MEDICAL MASTERCLASS

Emergency Medicine

Disclaimer

Although every effort has been made to ensure that drug doses and other information are presented accurately in this publication, the ultimate responsibility rests with the prescribing physician. Neither the publishers nor the authors can be held responsible for any consequences arising from the use of information contained herein. Any product mentioned in this publication should be used in accordance with the prescribing information prepared by the manufacturers.

The information presented in this publication reflects the opinions of its contributors and should not be taken to represent the policy and views of the Royal College of Physicians of London, unless this is specifically stated.

Every effort has been made by the contributors to contact holders of copyright to obtain permission to reproduce copyright material. However, if any have been inadvertently overlooked, the publisher will be pleased to make the necessary arrangements at the first opportunity.

Medical Masterclass

EDITOR-IN-CHIEF

John D. Firth DM FRCP
Consultant Physician and Nephrologist
Addenbrooke's Hospital
Cambridge

Emergency Medicine

EDITOR

Paul F. Jenkins MA MB BChir FRCP
Consultant Physician
Norfolk and Norwich Hospital
Norwich

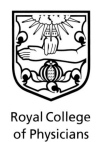

Royal College
of Physicians

Set and printed by Graphicraft Limited,
Hong Kong

ISBN: 1-86016-218-5 (this book)
ISBN: 1-86016-210-X (set)

Distribution Information:
Jerwood Medical Education Resource Centre
Royal College of Physicians of London
11 St. Andrews Place
Regent's Park
London NW1 4LE
United Kingdom
Tel: 0044 (0)207 935 1174 ext 422/490
Fax: 0044 (0)207 486 6653
Email: merc@rcplondon.ac.uk
Web: http://www.rcplondon.ac.uk/

Contents

List of contributors

C. Andrew Eynon BSc MBBS MRCP FFAEM
Specialist Registrar
John Radcliffe Hospital
Oxford

Paul F. Jenkins MA MB BChir FRCP
Consultant Physician
Norfolk and Norwich Hospital
Norwich

Carole M. Libetta MBChB MRCP FRCS(Ed)
Clinical Lecturer and Specialist Registrar
Emergency Department
Hope Hospital
Salford

Foreword

Since its foundation in 1518, the Royal College of Physicians has engaged in a wide range of activities dedicated to its overall aim of upholding and improving standards of medical practice. *Medical Masterclass* is one of the most innovative and ambitious educational resources the College has developed, and while it continues the tradition of pioneering and supporting high quality medicine, it also makes use of modern day technology by offering computer-assisted learning.

The MRCP(UK) examination is crucial to the progress of physicians through their training. Preparation is not only essential for success in the examination, but it is also important for the acquisition of requisite knowledge, skills and attitudes appropriate for further training. With a pass rate of about 40% at each sitting of the written papers, the exam is a challenge. The College wishes to encourage excellence, and with this in mind has produced *Medical Masterclass*, a comprehensive distance-learning package designed to help candidates with the preparation that is key to making the grade.

Medical Masterclass has been produced by the RCP's Education Department. It represents a formidable amount of work by Dr John Firth and his team of authors and editors. I congratulate our colleagues for this superb educational product and wholeheartedly recommend it as an invaluable MRCP(UK) study aid.

Professor Carol M. Black CBE
President of the Royal College of Physicians

Preface

Medical Masterclass comprises twelve paper-based modules, two CD-ROMs and a companion website. Its aim is to help doctors in their first few years of training to improve their medical skills and knowledge.

The twelve paper-based modules are divided as follows: two cover the scientific background to medicine, one is devoted to general clinical issues, one to emergency medicine and practical procedures, and eight cover the range of medical specialities. Medicine is often fairly straightforward when the diagnosis is clear, but patients rarely come to their doctor and say 'I've got Hodgkin's disease': they have lumps. The core material of each of the clinical specialities is defined by case presentations in the first part of each module: how do you approach the man who has lumps? Structured concise notes on specific diseases follow later. All practising doctors know that medicine is much more than knowing lots of facts about diseases: how do you tell someone they've got cancer? How do you decide when to stop treatment? Most medical texts say little about these issues: *Medical Masterclass* does not avoid them, nor does it talk in vague and abstract terms.

The two CD-ROMs each contain 30 interactive cases requiring diagnosis and treatment. The format is remarkably close to real life: you see the patient and are told the story; you have to decide how to investigate and treat; but you can't see all the results before you start to make decisions!

The companion website, which will be regularly updated, includes self-assessment questions and mock MRCP(UK) exam papers. How much do you know, and are you improving? You will see how your score compares with your previous attempts, and also how your performance compares with others who have logged on to the site.

The *Medical Masterclass* is produced by the Education Department of the Royal College of Physicians. It has been specifically designed to support candidates studying for the MRCP(UK) Examination (All Parts). I have no doubt that someone putting effort into learning through the *Medical Masterclass* would be in a strong position to impress the examiners.

John Firth
Editor-in-Chief

Acknowledgements

Medical Masterclass has been produced by a team. The names of those who have written and edited material are clearly indicated elsewhere, but without the efforts of many other people *Medical Masterclass* would not exist at all. These include Professor Lesley Rees and Mrs Winnie Wade from the Education Department of the Royal College of Physicians of London, who initiated the project; Dr Mike Stein and Dr Andy Robinson from Medschool.com and Blackwell Science respectively, who have enthusiastically supported it from the beginning; and Ms Filipa Maia and Ms Katherine Bowker, who have run the office with splendid efficiency and induced authors and editors to perform to a schedule rarely achieved. I and the whole of the team of editors and authors are immensely grateful to all of these people for the energy that they have poured into *Medical Masterclass* in various ways.

John Firth
Editor-in-Chief

Key features

We have created a range of icon boxes to help you identify key information and to make learning easier and more enjoyable. Here is a brief explanation:

Clinical pointer

This icon highlights important information to be noted.

Further information

This icon indicates the source of further information and reference.

Hints

This icon highlights useful hints, tips and mnemonics.

Key points

This icon is used to highlight points of particular importance.

Quote

This icon indicates useful or interesting citations from notable individuals, including well-known physicians.

Think about

This icon indicates what the reader should reflect on after having read a passage from the text.

Warning/Hazard

This icon is used to indicate common or important drug interactions, pitfalls of practical procedures, or when to take symptoms or signs particularly seriously.

Emergency Medicine

AUTHORS:
C.A. Eynon, P.F. Jenkins and C.M. Libetta

EDITOR:
P.F. Jenkins

EDITOR-IN-CHIEF:
J.D. Firth

1 Clinical presentations

1.1 Cardiac arrest

Case history

A 75-year-old man is found collapsed in bed on the ward after being admitted 3 days previously with an inferior myocardial infarction. You are called as a member of the cardiac arrest team and cardiorespiratory arrest is diagnosed.

Clinical approach

Three general points before discussing the details of cardiopulmonary resuscitation (CPR):
• Return of spontaneous circulation (ROSC) occurs in approximately 30% of in-hospital cardiac arrests but only 15% of patients survive to hospital discharge. Only 2% of out-of-hospital cardiac arrests survive to hospital discharge.
• Cardiorespiratory arrest is common to all causes of death, and CPR should be attempted only when there is a potentially reversible cause for the arrest. A decision not to attempt resuscitation should be clearly written in both the medical and the nursing notes and, ideally, should be discussed with the patient and/or relatives. This decision must be reviewed if clinical circumstances change [1].
• The practice of 'slow codes' or '... if he arrests, I would try one shock ...' is to be condemned.
In the case described, CPR has been deemed appropriate.

Management

Basic life support

The European Resuscitation Council guidelines for adult single-rescuer basic life support (BLS) are shown in Fig. 1 [2]. All members of a cardiac arrest team should be proficient in BLS.

 Cardiac output during closed-chest compressions ranges from a quarter to a third of normal. Diastolic arterial pressure and consequently coronary perfusion pressure fall rapidly after the first few minutes of CPR.

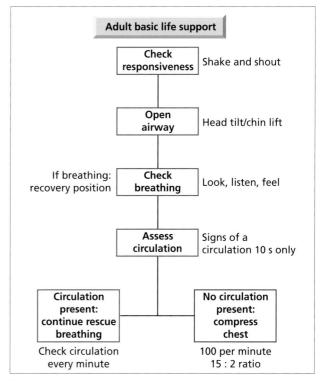

Fig. 1 European Resuscitation Council guidelines for adult basic life support. (From The 1998 European Resuscitation Council guidelines for adult single rescuer basic life support. A statement from the Working Group on Basic Life Support. *Resuscitation* 1998; 37: 67–80. © ERC. Published by Elsevier Science Ireland Ltd.)

Advanced life support

The European Resuscitation Council guidelines for adult advanced life support (ALS) are shown in Fig. 2 [3].

The defibrillator/monitor should be attached as soon as possible. Three primary categories of cardiac arrest rhythm are recognized:
1 ventricular fibrillation or pulseless ventricular tachycardia (VF/VT)
2 asystole
3 pulseless electrical activity (PEA).
If VF/VT is present, defibrillate ×3 as necessary. The first two shocks are given at 200 J in adults and the third at 360 J. Transthoracic impedance reduces with each shock such that each shock delivers more energy to the heart.

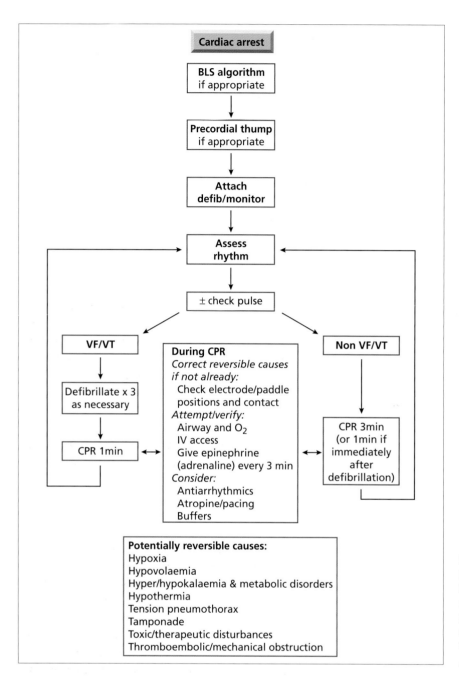

Fig. 2 European Resuscitation Council guidelines for adult advanced life support. BLS, basic life support; CPR, cardiopulmonary resuscitation. (From The 1998 European Resuscitation Council guidelines for adult advanced life support. A statement from the Working Group on Advanced Life Support. *Resuscitation* 1998; 37: 81–90. © ERC.)

Survival from cardiac arrest depends on the arrest rhythm.
• The survival rate for VF/VT is 10–15 times higher than for asystole or PEA.
• In VF/VT, survival correlates with time to defibrillation.
• Over 80% of patients resuscitated from VF/VT are resuscitated with one of the first three shocks.
• For asystole and PEA, ALS aims to maintain organ perfusion until remediable causes for the arrest can be sought and rectified.

Rescuer safety is paramount. All persons using a defibrillator should be fully trained in its use.

If the rhythm does not change post-defibrillation:
• A pulse check is unnecessary.
• If the first three shocks are unsuccessful, recommence CPR.
• Obtain and secure an airway and administer high-flow O_2. Obtain intravenous access.
• Give epinephrine (adrenaline) 1 mg i.v. every 3 minutes.
• Reassess the rhythm every minute and defibrillate as necessary.

If asystole/PEA is present:
• Recommence CPR.
• Obtain and secure an airway and administer high-flow O_2. Obtain intravenous access.
• Give epinephrine (adrenaline) 1 mg i.v. every 3 minutes.

• Assessing for potentially reversible causes is vitally important.

 Potentially reversible causes of asystole/PEA include:
• Hypoxia: ensure 100% O_2 is being administered, preferably via an endotracheal tube or laryngeal mask airway.
• Hypovolaemia: administer a rapid fluid bolus of 500–1000 mL 0.9% saline. Palpate for abdominal aortic aneurysm. Check for rectal bleeding.
• Hypo-/hyperkalaemia and metabolic disorders: check clinical history for clues. If known renal patient, presume hyperkalaemia and give 10 mL 10% $CaCl_2$ i.v.
• Hypothermia: the patient is never dead until they are warm and dead.
• Tension pneumothorax: consider especially in patients with pre-existing lung disease or if on a ventilator. Immediate needle decompression of the affected side is mandatory.
• Tamponade: diagnosis is difficult. There is nothing to lose by attempting pericardiocentesis.
• Toxins: including drug overdose. Check clinical history for clues.
• Pulmonary embolism (PE): always consider as a potential primary diagnosis.

The patient described in this case history was in ventricular fibrillation and was returned to sinus rhythm with a good cardiac output after the second defibrillation.

Further comments on the management of cardiac arrest

Basic life support

• BLS comprises initial assessment, maintenance of the airway, rescue breathing and closed-chest compression.
• The primary objective is to provide sufficient oxygenated blood to the brain and heart until definitive therapy can be applied and a spontaneous circulation reestablished.
• It is a holding method only but at least doubles the chances of survival if applied between the times of collapse and first defibrillation.

Advanced care

Airway management

Endotracheal intubation remains the gold standard, but the ease of insertion of laryngeal mask airways means that their use is increasing in the setting of cardiac arrest.

Vasopressors

Epinephrine (adrenaline) remains the first-line vasopressor for use in cardiac arrest, although it has not been shown to improve survival.

Antiarrhythmics

There is no clear evidence for the use of antiarrhythmics in cardiac arrest. Although atropine is of use for haemodynamically significant bradycardia, its use in asystole is based on limited data.

Buffers

Adequate ventilation and tissue perfusion is the best way to treat the combined metabolic and respiratory acidosis seen in cardiac arrest. In the specific cases of arrest associated with tricyclic antidepressant overdose, hyperkalaemia and pre-existing metabolic acidosis, giving sodium bicarbonate intravenously may be of benefit.

Pacing

External pacing of asystole has shown no clinical benefit. Pacing may be of occasional use for the treatment of ventricular standstill.

When to stop?

If ROSC does not occur promptly, consideration must be given to termination of the attempt:
• A delay of >5 min to start of BLS or of >30 min to defibrillation is associated with an extremely poor prognosis.
• In the absence of reversible factors, attempts to resuscitate non-VF/VT should be abandoned after 20 min.
• Hypothermia and the ingestion of cerebral depressants (sedatives, hypnotics, narcotics) provide some measure of cerebral protection.
• The presence of sepsis, disseminated cancer or major organ failure is associated with very poor outcome.
• Age itself is not an independent predictor for the success of resuscitation. Lower survival rates in the elderly reflect higher rates of comorbidity.

Relatives—in or out?

In many A&E Departments and Medical Admission Units it has become standard practice to allow relatives to observe resuscitation.
• The presence of family members during resuscitation efforts has been shown to aid the grieving process should resuscitation prove unsuccessful.

- Families should not be encouraged to enter the resuscitation room if they are reluctant.
- Relatives can only be allowed to observe resuscitation if there is a trained member of staff present whose sole responsibility is to support them; to have relatives watching, with no one to explain what is going on and attend to their needs, is asking for trouble.

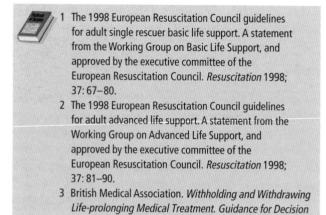

1 The 1998 European Resuscitation Council guidelines for adult single rescuer basic life support. A statement from the Working Group on Basic Life Support, and approved by the executive committee of the European Resuscitation Council. *Resuscitation* 1998; 37: 67–80.

2 The 1998 European Resuscitation Council guidelines for adult advanced life support. A statement from the Working Group on Advanced Life Support, and approved by the executive committee of the European Resuscitation Council. *Resuscitation* 1998; 37: 81–90.

3 British Medical Association. *Withholding and Withdrawing Life-prolonging Medical Treatment. Guidance for Decision Making.* London: BMJ Books, 1999.

1.2 Collapse with hypotension

Case history

You are called to A&E to see a woman aged 75 years who has been brought in by 'blue-light' ambulance. She has collapsed and has a systolic blood pressure of 60 mmHg. No history is available.

Clinical approach

The priorities are:
- Resuscitate (airway, breathing, circulation—ABC) and secure venous access.
- Examine the patient with a clear idea of the possible diagnoses (Table 1).
- Ask a colleague to enquire regarding any available history—ask ambulancemen, relatives or neighbours. When was the patient last seen? Is there any information about her past medical history?

Resuscitation and venous access

Regardless of the specific diagnosis, your priorities will be to correct any problem with airway, ventilation or

Table 1 Differential diagnosis of hypotensive collapse.

Common	Must consider	Other causes
Cardiovascular catastrophe: Myocardial infarction Pulmonary embolism	Aortic dissection	Addisonian crisis
	Tension pneumothorax	Hypothermia or hypothyroidism
Hypovolaemia (particularly gastrointestinal blood loss)	Fluid loss from other causes (e.g. profound diarrhoea in an elderly person living alone)	Pericardial disease with cardiac tamponade
A surgical cause—ruptured abdominal aortic aneurysm or a perforated viscus	Multiple problems— particularly in the elderly (e.g. acute viral infection, inadequate fluid intake and complicating myocardial infarction)	
Sepsis (pneumonia, septicaemia)		

circulation, to institute CPR if necessary and to obtain venous access.

Two large (grey) venflons should be inserted into the antecubital fossae. If this is not possible, then attempt femoral venous cannulation.

Central venous cannulation in the neck should not be attempted at this stage unless there is no alternative and then only by someone with experience of the technique. There are two reasons for saying this. First, other resuscitation measures may demand free access to the head and neck. Secondly, accessing the internal jugular or subclavian vein in a patient who is hypovolaemic is difficult and an iatrogenic pneumo- or haemothorax is not a good idea (Fig. 3).

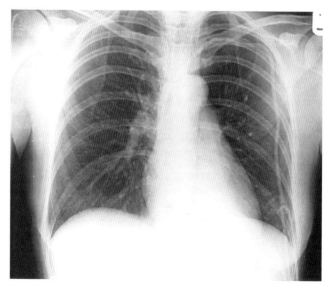

Fig. 3 Left subclavian line, iatrogenic left pneumothorax.

Examination

In assessing the patient with circulatory collapse:
- Accurate measurement of jugular venous pressure (JVP) is crucial. Measure in centimetres from the angle of Louis, angling the patient as necessary up or down until venous pulsation is seen. It is not good enough to settle for 'venous pressure not elevated'.
- If cardiac output is impaired, for whatever reason, there is often a marked cut-off peripherally between warm, dry skin and a cold, clammy feel. Run your hand down the patient's arm, starting from the shoulder and observe where the change occurs. If it is at mid forearm, cardiac output is severely compromised and if it is felt at the elbow, you should be very worried.
- Measurement of simple vital signs is essential: ensure that this is performed accurately. Temperature should be measured orally or rectally, axillary temperatures are totally unreliable. Pulse and blood pressure should be verified by medical staff and respiratory rate should be measured over 1 min, not guessed at.
- The absence of pyrexia does not exclude sepsis and this applies to the young as well as the elderly. Indeed, the severely septic patient may be hypothermic.
- Cultivate the technique of 'problem-solving' with your clinical examination when an abnormal physical sign leads you to seek other signs in a pathway that will narrow the differential diagnosis.

Immediate assessment of fluid balance is fundamental to management. Causes of hypotension include lack of circulating volume, circulatory pump (heart) failure or sepsis. In the latter situation a combination of peripheral vasodilatation, hypovolaemia and compromised myocardial function contribute to the abnormal haemodynamics.
- Do the physical signs suggest hypovolaemia with a low JVP and a postural fall (lying and sitting) in blood pressure?
- Is the JVP elevated as in heart failure, pulmonary embolus or with pericardial disease?
- Are the peripheries warm (usually in sepsis) or cold (as typically in cardiovascular collapse—see below)?

When examining a patient with circulatory collapse, continually run through the list of causes of hypotensive collapse shown in Table 1. Which of these is most likely? Pay particular attention to diagnoses that require specific treatments.

General

Are those few purpuric spots significant? (see *Infectious diseases*, Section 1.2).

Vital signs

Accurate measurement of pulse, blood pressure, degree of pulsus.paradoxus, temperature and respiratory rate are fundamental to establishing the diagnosis, and the task of

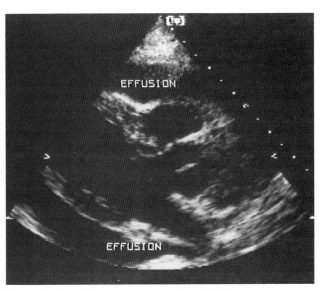

Fig. 4 An echocardiogram of a large pericardial effusion.

recording these vital signs should not be delegated to a junior nurse.

Cardiovascular

Can you feel the left radial pulse as well as the right? If not, consider aortic dissection.

Listen for murmurs and additional heart sounds. Try to decide if an obvious third heart sound relates to the left ventricle or to the right. Mitral valve regurgitation or a traumatic ventricular septal defect can complicate acute myocardial infarction and precipitate catastrophic heart failure (see *Cardiology*, Section 1.7). Also, always consider the possibility of subacute bacterial endocarditis when a murmur is discovered, looking specifically for confirmatory signs of this condition (see *Cardiology*, Section 1.13).

It is easy to overlook the possibility of a pericardial effusion (Fig. 4) but the diagnostic signs of pulsus paradoxus (which must be measured with a sphygmomanometer) and elevation of the venous pressure with inspiration (Kussmaul's sign) should be a part of your routine examination (see *Cardiology*, Section 1.8).

Respiratory

Consider tension pneumothorax, which can present with circulatory collapse or cardiac arrest. The features are:
- the chest often looks asymmetrical, with the affected side 'blown up'
- tracheal deviation
- mediastinal shift
- the affected side of chest is silent.

If this is the diagnosis, immediately insert a venflon into the chest in the second intercostal, space midclavicular line or midaxillary line in the axilla.

Bronchial breathing associated with dullness to percussion in the hypotensive, septic patient may indicate community-acquired pneumonia—but beware, aspiration pneumonia complicates many causes of hypotensive collapse and the physical signs (and the chest radiograph) can be identical.

Abdominal

Feel deliberately for an abdominal aortic aneurysm and look for bruising in the flanks. Look for signs of peritonism or intestinal obstruction and remember basic observations; is there abdominal distension, is there visible peristalsis and is there a femoral hernia?

Rectal examination is mandatory to exclude melaena.

Neurological

Carefully assess conscious level and record your observations using the Glasgow Coma Scale (GCS). Look for abnormal focal neurological signs, pupillary changes, abnormalities of ocular movement and disordered respiratory rhythm which may point to brain-stem pathology (see Section 1.26, p. 76).

The hypotensive patient who is unconscious:
Note the question of the chicken and the egg: which came first? It is much more likely that hypotension has caused coma by inducing cerebral damage than that a primary intracerebral process has caused circulatory collapse.

One of the arts of clinical examination is to make an observation which leads you to seek associated signs, which then leads to a diagnosis, e.g. is the third heart sound accompanied by a parasternal heave and elevation in venous pressure, perhaps with an accentuated 'a' wave? If so, the evidence for a major PE is strong.

Approach to investigations and management

Investigations

Blood tests

An immediate BM stix estimation of sugar is mandatory in this as in other emergency situations.

Basic haematological and biochemical tests are required and should be requested urgently: haemoglobin, mean corpuscular volume (MCV), mean corpuscular haemoglobin concentration (MCHC), absolute and differential white cell count, urea and electrolytes, liver function tests, blood sugar and cardiac enzymes.

Blood cultures (and sometimes other cultures, e.g. urine, cerebrospinal fluid (CSF) are mandatory, regardless of your initial suspicion of sepsis, unless another confident diagnosis can be made immediately, e.g. myocardial infarction.

Pulse oximetry can be unreliable in patients who are hypotensive: measurement of arterial blood gases is essential to check O_2 tension and pH, looking for hypoxia and acidosis in particular.

Electrocardiogram

A 12-lead ECG should be done immediately: look for a myocardial infarction pattern, and also for ischaemic change and abnormal rate and rhythm. In this setting, old traces are unlikely to be available, so be aware of subtle changes that may aid diagnosis, e.g. the tall P wave of acute pulmonary hypertension, or small voltage complexes in standard leads which may be seen in the presence of pericardial fluid.

Radiology

Most would consider that a chest radiograph in the emergency medical patient is an extension of the clinical examination. The chest film can provide much information; it will aid decisions regarding fluid balance as well as excluding many intrathoracic causes for severe hypotension.

Abdominal radiographs are requested too frequently: they are useful only in the case of perforation of a viscus or in intestinal obstruction and should be ordered only when these are plausible diagnoses. This is important because abdominal films are difficult to take with a portable X-ray machine and transporting the hypotensive patient to the radiography department has to be a calculated decision, undertaken only when it is likely to aid management.

Other tests

Examination findings may demand additional investigations—thyroid function tests, an abdominal ultrasound, a thoracic CT scan if aortic dissection is suspected (see Section 1.3, pp. 11, 13) or CT angiography of the chest in a compromised patient with suspected PE (see Section 1.8, pp. 29–30).

Management

Be obsessional in your assessment of intravascular volume. Is the patient hypovolaemic or is there another reason for hypotension? If you are unclear about this, get help and/or measure the central venous pressure (CVP). It is not a good idea to give a fluid challenge to someone who is in heart failure.

Be wary with central lines—do not over-interpret the information that they can provide: right-sided cardiac pressures reveal only part of the picture. It is possible to have a normal or high right atrial pressure at a time when left ventricular filling is inadequate, e.g. with major embolus.

Any of the conditions listed in Table 1 will require rapid specific treatment:
- myocardial infarction (see Section 1.3 and *Cardiology*, Section 1.5)
- pulmonary embolism (see *Cardiology*, Sections 1.8 and 1.9)
- tension pneumothorax (see Section 1.10, p. 36)
- gastrointestinal haemorrhage (see *Gastroenterology*, Section 1.3).

Arrange for urgent surgical consultation if appropriate, e.g. if the main problem seems to be abdominal. You cannot afford to waste time with someone who is desperately ill—resuscitation and decisions about investigation (urgent CT scan of the abdomen?) or laparotomy should be made concurrently.

Issues of importance to all patients are described below.

Oxygen

Give high-flow O_2, except to the very few patients who retain CO_2.

Fluid replacement

Appropriate fluids should be given to the hypovolaemic patient.

If there is evidence of acute blood loss then blood should be transfused. An emergency cross match should be available within 20–30 min, but if fluid replacement is more urgent than this then colloid solutions can be given or, in extreme circumstances, O negative blood.

When there is no evidence of blood loss, intravenous replacement will consist of colloid or crystalloid solutions: in most cases 0.9% saline (normal saline) will be appropriate.

Insert a urinary catheter to monitor output.

Resuscitation should be swift! There is no merit in resuscitating more slowly than is possible.

If you are confident that a patient is hypovolaemic, then give intravenous fluids quickly until the circulation is restored. The rules are simple:
- Look at the JVP or measure the CVP.
- Record blood pressure, lying and sitting.
- Give 1–2 L of colloid/0.9% saline quickly, as fast as access will allow.

- Repeat inspection of JVP/CVP and blood pressure.
- If JVP/CVP and blood pressure are restored, stop rapid infusions.
- If JVP/CVP and blood pressure are *not* restored, give another 1 L quickly.
- Repeat the process until circulation is restored.

If the patient remains hypotensive when intravascular volume has been restored, consider:
- The need for an additional fluid challenge, but do not induce fluid overload and pulmonary oedema: very few hearts work better if the CVP is pushed above 8–10 cm.
- Inotropes can be used if there is circulatory pump failure and vasoconstricting drugs may be necessary if vasodilatation is a part of the pathological process, as for example in sepsis.

If the patient does not improve rapidly following initial resuscitation, now is the time for comprehensive haemodynamic measurements: a pulmonary artery flotation catheter will allow measurement of left-sided cardiac pressures, cardiac output, systemic vascular resistance and objective indices of myocardial function. However, before escalating treatment in this way, the appropriateness of intensive care for the individual patient must be discussed and ratified (see Sections 1.5, p. 21 and 1.10, p. 37).

Antibiotics

'If in doubt dish them out'—it is better to err on the side of antibiotic prescription. One or two doses of broad-spectrum antibiotics will do no harm, but failure to recognize and to treat sepsis promptly can be catastrophic. Remember:
- Sepsis can present atypically.
- Always take blood cultures before prescribing antibiotics.

When managing the hypotensive patient:
- Airway, breathing, circulation.
- Give high-flow O_2 (unless CO_2 retainer).
- Is the patient hypovolaemic or is there an alternative reason for hypotension?
- If hypovolaemic, give the correct fluid quickly.
- Is specific treatment indicated for the particular primary pathology?
- If still hypotensive, proceed to invasive haemodynamic measurement, inotropic and/or vasoconstricting drugs as indicated.
- The indication for intensive care must be clear and appropriate for the individual patient.

1 Webb AR, Shapiro MJ, Singer M, Suter PM. *Oxford Textbook of Critical Care*. Oxford: Oxford Medical Publications, 1999.
2 Shoemaker WC, Ayres SM, Grenvik A, Holbrook PR. *Textbook of Critical Care*, 3rd edn. Philadelphia: WB Saunders, 1995.

1.3 Central chest pain

Case history

A 57-year-old businessman presents with a history of severe central crushing chest pain of 1 hour's duration. This followed a stressful business meeting and his colleagues have brought him to A&E where you are asked to see him.

Clinical approach

Prioritize your actions: resuscitate as necessary, give high-flow O_2 and obtain adequate venous access. There are four key areas to explore:

1 Is he still in pain? If so, analgesics should be administered and opiates may well be necessary.

2 What are the haemodynamic findings? Are his pulse, blood pressure (including paradox) and JVP normal? If he is breathless, do the findings suggest heart failure or pulmonary embolism?

3 Is the pain cardiac? This will be your main diagnostic concern; an immediate decision will be required regarding the need for thrombolysis (see below), but it is just as important to recognize continuing cardiac pain with no evidence of infarction. The acute coronary syndrome indicates that cardiac muscle is at risk and prompt medication with aspirin, heparin, β-blockade and perhaps nitrates should be instituted.

4 What is the differential diagnosis? The main differentials are shown in Table 2. As a priority, consider life-threatening conditions other than myocardial infarction/acute coronary syndrome, e.g. aortic dissection or a PE.

 PE typically causes pleuritic pain but can present with symptoms of myocardial ischaemia.

 If a firm diagnosis cannot be established on the basis of history, examination and immediate tests then your default position must be to assume that the patient has cardiac ischaemia.

Table 2 Differential diagnosis of central chest pain.

Common	Must consider	Other causes
Myocardial infarction/acute coronary syndrome	Aortic dissection	Pericarditis
	Pulmonary embolism	Referred from
Oesophagitis		abdomen, e.g.
Musculoskeletal		peptic ulcer
Unknown		

History of presenting problem

A detailed description of the chest pain is required.

When, where and how?

Ask specific questions:
• When did the pain start?
• Were you in bed, sitting at your desk, walking upstairs, stressed or angry?
• Where did you feel the pain? Ask for the specific site of the pain.
• How did the pain start? Suddenly? Coming on over a period of time?

 Ischaemic cardiac pain is typically exacerbated by exercise or emotion, but can occur at rest, when the implications are more serious. It tends to be felt in the middle of the chest, does not start suddenly, but builds up over a few minutes.

Nature of the pain

Classic cardiac pain is described as 'like a heavy weight', '... as if I was being squeezed in a vice' or '... it was as if someone was sitting on my chest'. Notice the patient's gestures; if he makes a fist over the centre of his chest when asked to describe the pain, this is typical of cardiac ischaemia.

Ask specifically:
• Was the pain frightening?
• Were you in a cold sweat?
• Did you think you were going to die?
• Did you feel nauseated or vomit?
These features are all suggestive of cardiac pain.

Radiation

Cardiac pain classically radiates to the shoulders and down one or both arms. However, radiation to the mandible or lower teeth is even more specific and you should enquire for this feature directly.

Duration of the pain

Ischaemic cardiac pain lasts for minutes or hours; it does not disappear after a few seconds.

Clues to other diagnoses

Are there any features which might suggest one of the conditions listed in Table 2?

Aortic dissection

The pain typically comes on suddenly, is usually sited in the back or radiates through to the back, and is often described as 'tearing' in nature.

Musculoskeletal pain

Sometimes local tenderness is present (but be wary, this can be a feature of embolic pleurisy) and sometimes the pain can be reproduced by thoracic spinal movements. Often the patient will report that discomfort is exacerbated by particular movements or a particular body position.

Oesophageal pain

Acid or an unpleasant taste in the mouth may accompany pain of oesophageal origin but the distinction from cardiac pain can be very difficult.

Pericarditis

Pericardial pain is typically described as being 'tight', but with pleuritic features as well, and there may be a history of a preceding 'flu-like illness (see *Cardiology*, Section 2.6.1).

Pulmonary embolism

The varied presentations of PE, many of them atypical and not backed by classic examination findings and investigations make for a potentially difficult diagnosis (see Section 1.8, pp. 29–32).

PE may present with ischaemic cardiac pain, and indeed there may be ischaemic changes on the ECG which relate to the left ventricle rather than the right. This is because the sudden increase in after-load on the right ventricle may result in myocardial ischaemia (or even secondary myocardial infarction), particularly if the patient has abnormal coronary arteries. Moreover, depending on the relative distribution of coronary artery disease, it may be the left ventricle that suffers most. This is a classic diagnostic trap.

Risk factors

Coronary artery disease is more likely in a middle-aged or elderly male smoker who is diabetic and who has a family history of premature ischaemic heart disease, hypertension or hypercholesterolaemia. How many of these factors apply to this patient? (But beware, myocardial infarction does occur in the absence of recognized risk factors.)

Examination

What does the patient look like? Are they well, ill, very ill or nearly dead? If they are cold, clammy and hypotensive, the diagnosis is serious and a cardiovascular cause for their pain is likely. If, on the other hand, they are calm, smiling and reading a book, they are unlikely to be in the throes of a myocardial infarction.

The most important points to consider are:
- Is there any evidence of heart failure; an elevated JVP, dyspnoea (particularly when lying flat) or typical chest signs?
- Is there a pericardial or pleural rub, indicating pericarditis or pleurisy, respectively?
- Is the pain exacerbated by movement when a musculoskeletal cause may be responsible?
- Is the pulse weak at the left wrist or the blood pressure unequal in the arms or is there an aortic regurgitant murmur? These are signs associated with aortic dissection.
- Anxiety. Be wary of diagnosing anxiety as the cause of chest pain. Anxiety is a common and totally understandable accompaniment of organic chest discomfort.

Approach to investigations and management

When seeing a patient with chest pain, ask yourself:
- Is this cardiac pain?
- Is thrombolysis indicated?
- If not cardiac, is there an alternative life-threatening condition, e.g. PE or aortic dissection?
- Do I need senior help?
Be safe and not sorry: assume an acute coronary syndrome unless you can make a confident alternative diagnosis.

Investigations

Electrocardiogram

Organize this immediately; do not delay while you take a history from the patient. The priority is to detect ECG evidence of myocardial infarction (Fig. 5) and the ECG criteria for thrombolytic therapy (Table 3). Keep the 'door to needle time' as short as possible.

The ECG should be repeated after half an hour and at any time if there is recurrence of pain. Do not miss the opportunity for thrombolysis.

Look also for features of pericarditis. The typical ECG changes are of peaked 'T' waves and S-T segments, which are elevated and concave upwards, but there is another appearance which can help with the diagnosis. The isoelectric line on the ECG is the T-P interval and in acute pericarditis there is sometimes depression of the P-R interval, which follows (Fig. 6).

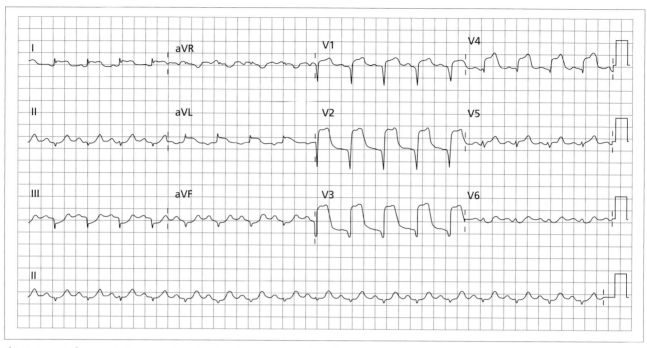

Fig. 5 An ECG of acute anterior myocardial infarction with early Q wave formation.

Table 3 ECG criteria for thrombolysis.

1 mm or more S-T segment elevation in two or more standard ECG leads
2 mm or more elevation in two or more contiguous praecordial leads (in typical infarct pattern)
New left bundle branch block

Blood tests

Check full blood count, cardiac enzymes, renal and liver function tests, blood sugar and cholesterol levels.

Chest radiograph

Measure heart size, exclude pulmonary oedema and look for the widened mediastinum of aortic dissection.

Management

Myocardial infarction

See *Cardiology*, Sections 1.5 and 2.1.3.

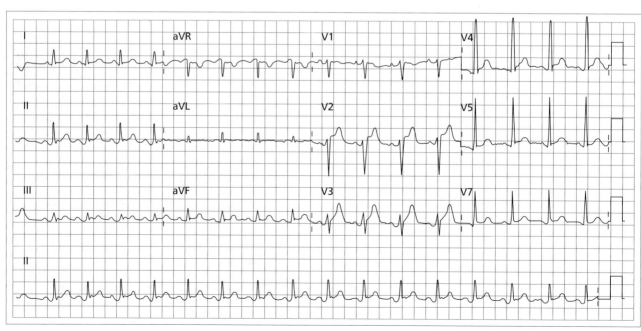

Fig. 6 An ECG of acute pericarditis; the S-T segment changes are obvious but note also the depressed P-R interval shown especially in leads II and aVF.

Table 4 Contraindications to thrombolysis. The greater the area of myocardium in jeopardy the greater the benefit from thrombolysis.

Cerebrovascular accident/peptic ulcer/gastrointestinal bleed within the preceding 3 months
Surgery or trauma within the preceding 2 weeks
Blood pressure more than 200/110
In pregnant or puerperal patients
If there is identified pulmonary cavitation
If duration of symptoms is more than 12 h (12–24 h if pain is still present)
Great caution in diabetic retinopathy or if heavy vaginal bleeding

THROMBOLYSIS

Thrombolytic therapy is one of the most important advances in medical treatment of the past two decades and should be administered as soon as possible after the confirmation of myocardial infarction by diagnostic ECG changes. Trials have indicated that patients with ECG criteria shown in Table 3 benefit from thrombolysis.

If there are no contraindications to thrombolysis (Table 4), streptokinase is the agent most commonly given, but there is evidence that tissue-type plasminogen activator (tpa) may be superior in anterior myocardial infarction when symptoms have been present for less than 4 h; tpa should always be used if streptokinase has been administered at any time in the past and in patients whose systolic blood pressure is less than 100 mmHg [1, 2].

ASPIRIN

Aspirin improves survival in myocardial infarction and should be given immediately.

β-BLOCKERS

A recent review of randomized controlled studies indicates that treatment with β-blockers postinfarction continued long term prevents around 12 deaths each year for every 1000 patients treated. Treatment should start early but (contrary to previous advice) initial intravenous therapy appears not to confer additional benefit [3].

The acute coronary syndrome

See *Cardiology*, Sections 1.5, 2.1.2 and 2.1.3.

If the history suggests cardiac pain but ECG evidence of myocardial infarction is absent, repeat the ECG in 30 min and at regular intervals thereafter if pain persists. Constantly question the need for thrombolysis. In this situation, pain indicates the presence of cardiac muscle at risk. It is possible to quantify the risk according to whether ECG changes (of S-T segment depression and/or T wave inversion) and/or elevation of cardiac troponin are present [4].

Treatment is mandatory and urgent:
• Aspirin is of proven benefit in reducing myocardial infarction and death and should be administered immediately [1, 2].
• β-Blockers should be given in unstable angina if tolerated.
• Heparin. Patients should be heparinized: low-molecular-weight heparin may be superior to unfractionated [5].
• Nitrates. All patients with unstable angina should receive nitrates; commence with sublingual buccal Suscard and progress to an intravenous preparation if pain persists.
• Calcium antagonists are indicated in variant angina and if β-blockers cannot be tolerated. A rate-limiting agent such as diltiazem should be used.
• Glycoprotein 2b, 3a receptor antagonists. The role of these agents is being assessed and, at the moment, their main indication appears to be plaque stabilization in the patient who requires angiography and who is a potential candidate for revascularization procedures (but see recent National Service Framework report).

Aortic dissection

If dissection is suspected, the definitive investigations are either computerized tomography (CT) (Fig. 7) or transoesophageal echocardiography (Fig. 8): whichever is most readily available should be used.

In proximal aortic dissection the prognosis is poor with medical management and surgery should be considered urgently.

Pericarditis

A therapeutic trial of aspirin or other non-steroidal anti-inflammatory drugs (NSAIDs) can sometimes help

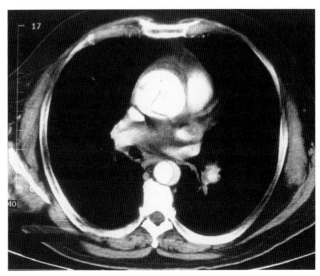

Fig. 7 A mediastinal CT scan showing the classical appearances of aortic dissection: note the 'tennis-ball' appearance in the ascending and descending aorta.

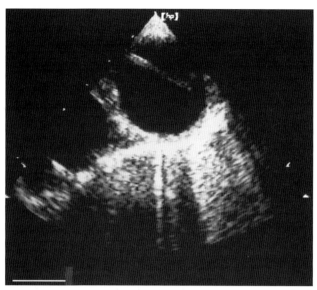

1 Risk of myocardial infarction and death during treatment with low-dose aspirin and intravenous heparin in men with unstable coronary artery disease. The RISC Group. *Lancet* 1990; 336: 827–830.
2 Wallentin LC. Aspirin (75 mg/day) after an episode of unstable coronary artery disease: long-term effects on the risk for myocardial infarction occurrence of severe angina and the need for revascularization. *J Am Coll Cardiol* 1991; 18: 1587–1593.
3 Freemantle N, Clelland J, Young P, Mason J, Harrison J. β-blockade after myocardial infarction: systematic review and metaregression analysis. *BMJ* 1999; 318: 1730–1737.
4 Lindahl B, Toss H, Siegbatin A, Venge P, Wallentin L. Markers of myocardial damage and inflammation in relation to long-term mortality in unstable coronary artery disease. FRISC Study Group. *N Engl J Med* 2000; 343: 1139–1147.
5 Cohen M, Blaber R, Demers C *et al.* Essence Trial. *J Thromb Thrombolysis* 1997; 4: 271–274.

Fig. 8 Transoesophageal echocardiogram showing the flap of dissection in the aorta.

in diagnosing pericarditis; relief of pericarditic pain commonly accrues within 20 min (see *Cardiology*, Section 2.6.1).

Oesophageal pain

Oesophageal discomfort can sound remarkably like cardiac pain and a therapeutic trial of antacid may be useful diagnostically. Remember, however, that nitrates can relieve oesophageal pain—although not usually as promptly as they improve angina pectoris.

Inevitably, there will be some situations in which it is impossible to decide between oesophageal and cardiac aetiology and in these situations your fall-back position must be to 'consider it cardiac until proved otherwise'. Deal with the situation as if it were the acute coronary syndrome.

'I do not know the diagnosis'

Be honest with yourself and with the patient. The fact that you do not know the diagnosis does not mean that you have 'failed': the diagnosis may be impossible to make. Your approach should be to consider the major diagnoses we have discussed. Therapeutic trials may aid diagnostically, but the default position will be to consider the most serious potential conditions and treat appropriately until further evidence has secured the diagnosis.

 It is better to overtreat for a few hours if the patient leaves the Emergency Room head first rather than feet first.

1.4 Tachyarrythmia

Case histories

You are the physician on acute medical intake one Monday afternoon when you receive a call from the Medical Admissions Unit informing you that two patients have just arrived, both with heart rates in excess of 150 beats/min. One woman is 25 years of age and is complaining of palpitation; the other patient, also female, is in her seventies and has central chest pain as well as palpitation.

Clinical approach

Immediate priorities

When dealing with any patient with tachyarrythmia the immediate priorities are:
• Assess accompanying symptoms, e.g. cardiac pain or breathlessness.
• Check haemodynamic status: is there evidence of low output—cold peripheries, hypotension? Is there evidence of pulmonary oedema?

If symptoms are present, or if there is haemodynamic compromise, then immediate correction of the rhythm disturbance is mandatory provided you are certain that the rapid heart rate is a primary and not a secondary or agonal phenomenon, e.g. in sinus tachycardia complicating a myocardial infarction with left ventricular failure. Examine a 12-lead ECG as soon as possible.

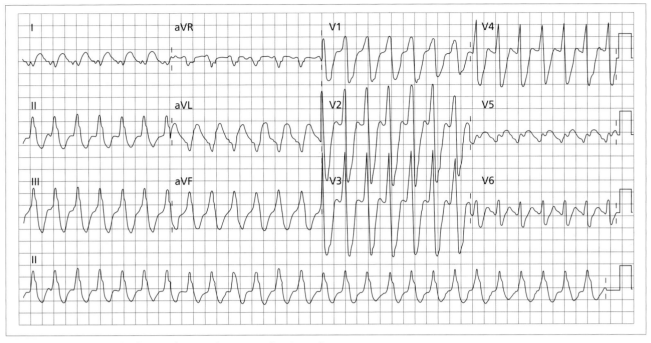

Fig. 9 Ventricular tachycardia showing dissociated P waves and QRS complexes.

Tachydysrhythmia—how fast do you need to act?
If your patient has a normal blood pressure, is not cold and clammy and does not have chest pain, you have time to think before you choose your preferred management.

'Milk' the ECG

Specific questions to ask:
• Are the QRS complexes narrow (less than 120 ms in duration) or broad (120 ms or more)?
• Broad-complex tachycardia is VT (Fig. 9) until proved otherwise.
• Attempt to differentiate ventricular and supraventricular rhythms using the guidelines below.

• Broad-complex tachycardia is VT until proved otherwise.
• It is important to have a low threshhold of suspicion for VT, which often requires early direct current (DC) cardioversion to prevent cardiac decompensation.

Examine previous records

If previous records are available, look through these quickly:
• Have there been episodes of tachydysrhythmia in the past and, if so, what was the final interpretation of the rhythm disturbance?
• Is there documentary evidence of structural heart problems, e.g. valve disease or cardiomyopathy?

• Can you find documented echocardiographic evidence of left ventricular function or any record of ischaemic heart disease?
• Is there evidence of an innate electrical abnormality, e.g. of the classical accessory pathways of the Wolff–Parkinson–White or the Lown–Ganong–Levine syndromes?

Seek out previous ECGs. These can provide vital information: traces obtained in sinus rhythm and during previous episodes of tachydysrhythmia can both be very useful.

History of the presenting problem

It is often difficult to ascertain the duration of the abnormal rhythm from the history. If atrial fibrillation (or atrial flutter) has been present for more than 48 h, there is a significant risk of systemic embolus if acute cardioversion to sinus rhythm is undertaken [1]. Be circumspect before attempting cardioversion, either electrical or with drugs, in the patient presenting with these rhythms. If they have been present for longer than 48 h, anticoagulants should be commenced and elective cardioversion should be considered after 4 weeks.

Details of previous episodes of tachydysrhythmia or of premorbid heart disease are vitally important: tachydysrhythmia in someone who has suffered a myocardial infarction or who has a cardiomyopathy is very likely to be due to VT.

Examination

Record vital signs accurately: compromised haemodynamic findings demand prompt treatment of the dysrhythmia. Key issues are:
- Rate.
- Rhythm—atrial fibrillation is the commonest cause of an irregular rhythm, although it may be difficult to ascertain irregularity clinically when the heart rate is high.
- Peripheral perfusion.
- Blood pressure.
- JVP—cannon waves indicate dissociation of atrial and ventricular contractions and their presence strongly suggests VT. Flutter waves can sometimes be seen in the neck; although a difficult physical sign, they are diagnostic of atrial flutter.
- Evidence of pulmonary oedema.

Contrary to popular belief, abnormal haemodynamic findings do not necessarily indicate a ventricular source of the dysrhythmia. VT can be tolerated for hours with no evidence of compromised cardiac output if myocardial function is good, whereas even a relatively slow supraventricular tachycardia (SVT) can be devastating in the presence of ischaemic or other heart disease, e.g. patients with hypertrophic obstructive cardiomyopathy characteristically tolerate atrial fibrillation very badly.

 When making your diagnosis of the type of tachyarrythmia, do not be influenced by haemodynamic findings.

Approach to investigations and management

Investigations

Information from the ECG

QRS COMPLEXES WIDENED (MORE THAN 120 MS IN DURATION) [2,3]

Essentially, the diagnosis is either VT or SVT with bundle branch block. Many ECG criteria and algorithms have been published as aids to differentiating these two possibilities, but they often rely on appearances that are difficult to interpret, particularly in the Emergency Room!

A diagnosis of VT can be made reliably in most cases by employing a few simple criteria:
- Atrioventricular (A-V) dissociation is the most reliable criterion for VT (see Fig. 9). Remember that the occasional 'blip' on the ECG is usually artefact, but if there are more QRS complexes than P waves this is 100% diagnostic of VT. Caution, though, atrial and ventricular

Table 5 Predictive value of QRS complex width in diagnosing ventricular tachycardia (VT) [2].

QRS width in seconds	Percentage of cases of VT
≤0.12	14
>0.12 to ≤0.14	43
>0.14 to ≤0.16	100
>0.16 to ≤0.18	100
>0.18	100

association can occur in VT if there is retrograde conduction through the A-V node.
- Capture beats and fusion beats are useful indicators of VT. A capture beat is a normal, usually (but not always) narrow, QRS complex surrounded by wide complexes and represents the triggering of ventricular depolarization by the regular atrial activity continuing between abnormal ventricular complexes. A fusion beat arises when a capture beat simultaneously depolarizes the ventricles with discharge from the abnormal ventricular focus; this leads to a wide, bizarre complex differing from the QRS complexes surrounding it. Both phenomena are rare occurrences but their presence usually secures the diagnosis of VT, although they have been reported rarely in the Wolff–Parkinson–White syndrome and in SVT with bundle branch block.
- The wider the QRS complexes are, the more likely they are to originate from a ventricular focus (Table 5).
- 'Concordance' is present if the QRS complexes have the same morphology across the chest leads. The pattern may be all positive or all negative. The presence of concordance, either positive or negative, is a reliable pointer to VT.
- Extreme left axis deviation and/or a definite axis shift in the dysrhythmia compared with previous ECGs in sinus rhythm are strong indicators of VT.
- Note one rare situation: antidromic conduction (down the bundle of Kent) in the WPW syndrome can produce a wide QRS complex tachycardia which demands particular treatment.

 Why is broad-complex tachycardia regarded as VT until proved otherwise?
- Wrongly diagnosing SVT is potentially disastrous: verapamil in VT is likely to cause severe and prolonged hypotension or even cardiac arrest.
- Manoeuvres to correct VT, on the other hand, are unlikely to cause further compromise in the patient with SVT.

QRS COMPLEXES NARROW (120 MS OR LESS IN DURATION)

The rhythm is very likely to be of supraventricular origin although rare forms of VT can manifest with narrow complexes. Questions to ask are:

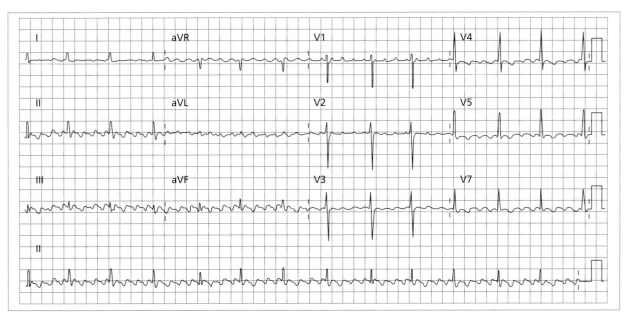

Fig. 10 Atrial flutter with 4 : 1 A-V block.

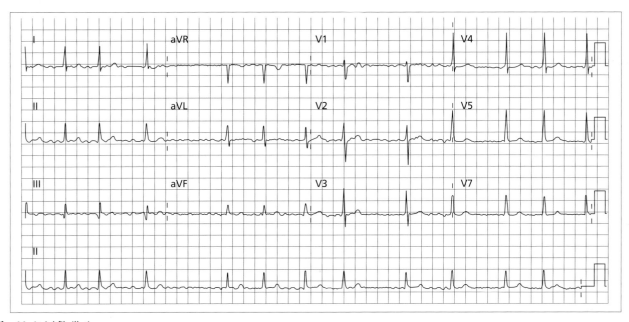

Fig. 11 Atrial fibrillation.

• Are the complexes regular? If so, what is the association of P waves to the QRS complexes? Is there evidence for 2 : 1 or 3 : 1 A-V block, etc.?

• What is the ventricular rate? If it is exactly 150/min (or nearly so) atrial flutter with 2 : 1 block is a real possibility, similarly 100/min with 3 : 1 block and 75/min with 4 : 1. The classical 'saw-tooth' pattern of atrial depolarization is diagnostic (Fig. 10).

• If the rhythm is irregular, search for atrial electrical activity. If this is present, paroxysmal atrial tachycardia or atrial flutter with variable A-V block is likely.

• Sometimes, atrial fibrillation may appear to have organized atrial activity but the typical hectic appearance of the QRS complexes usually leaves little doubt as to the true nature of the rhythm (Fig. 11).

Management

Adenosine

Adenosine, a purine nucleoside, is highly efficient at blocking the A-V node. Its action lasts for seconds only and it is not negatively inotropic.

It is contraindicated only in asthmatic patients and in those with a high degree of A-V block (second- or third-degree heart block). However, be cautious if dipyridamole is being taken as this drug potentiates the effect of adenosine.

Adenosine has revolutionized the management of tachydysrhythmia, not only by its ability to terminate SVTs induced by re-entrant phenomena, but also as a diagnostic tool in broad-complex tachycardia in helping to uncover the presence of atrial flutter and sometimes in confirming the presence of atrial fibrillation.

Adenosine should be administered as follows: start with a rapid bolus of 6 mg (which terminated the re-entrant SVT of the 25-year-old woman described above), moving to boluses of 9 mg and 12 mg if necessary. Each bolus should be followed immediately by a flush of saline into a large vein. Larger boluses of adenosine may be successful if this regimen has failed, but expert advice should be sought under these circumstances.

Adenosine is unlikely to be successful in terminating atrial flutter and atrial fibrillation.

Broad-complex tachycardia

The algorithm shown in Fig. 12 is intended to guide management, not to differentiate VT from SVT in all cases. If there is doubt, the default position is to diagnose VT and to treat accordingly [2, 3].

 If the patient is haemodynamically unstable, DC cardioversion should be undertaken without delay, regardless of whether the rhythm is ventricular or supraventricular.

DRUG TREATMENT OF BROAD-COMPLEX TACHYCARDIA

Lidocaine (lignocaine)
Lidocaine (50–100 mg as i.v. bolus, followed by infusion at 4 mg/min for 30 min; 2 mg/min for 2 h; then 1 mg/min) is the drug of first choice for VT as it is the safest in terms of side effects and adverse reactions.

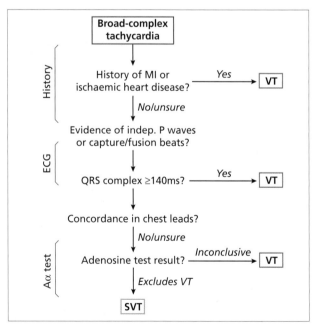

Fig. 12 Algorithm to aid decision-making in broad-complex tachycardia [2]. MI, myocardial infarction; SUT, supraventricular tachycardia; VT, ventricular tachycardia.

Second-line agents
Either sotalol (20–60 mg i.v. over 2–3 min, repeated if necessary after 10 min) or procainamide (500–600 mg over 25–30 min, followed by infusion at a rate of 2–6 mg/min) can be used.

Flecainide
This drug has a documented 55% cardioversion rate in trials but its pro-arrhythmic and hypotensive side effect rate of 25% makes it unacceptable for routine use.

 Management of broad-complex tachycardia:
- In the haemodynamically stable patient, give one antiarrhythmic agent.
- If this is unsuccessful in restoring normal rhythm, it will be safer to move to DC cardioversion rather than administering additional antiarrhythmic drugs and risk hypotension or other adverse effects.
- This approach may be modified if expert help is to hand.

The woman in her seventies with chest pain had a history of ischaemic heart disease and her VT was treated with cardioversion followed by sotalol.

Narrow-complex tachycardia

ATRIAL FIBRILLATION

The options are:
- DC cardioversion if the patient is compromised haemodynamically or has cardiac pain.
- Digitalize to control ventricular rate. Digoxin should usually be given orally (1.0–1.5 mg in divided doses over 24 h), but can be given by intravenous injection in emergency (0.25–0.5 mg over 10–20 min, repeated after 4–8 h to total loading dose 0.5–1.0 mg).
- Consider heparinization in all cases because of the risk of atrial thrombus formation (see above), a risk enhanced if sinus rhythm returns following DC or medical cardioversion, with drugs such as flecainide (50 mg bd p.o., maximum 300 mg daily; alternatively 2 mg/kg i.v. over 10–30 min [maximum 150 mg], followed if necessary by infusion). Amiodarone can be given orally and a large single dose (30 mg/kg) can be highly effective [4] as an alternative to the traditional loading dose of 200–400 mg tds for 3–7 days. Alternatively, amiodarone can be given i.v. (5 mg/kg) over 20–120 min but this needs to be into a central vein (maximum 1.2 g in 24 h).

ATRIAL FLUTTER

DC cardioversion should be considered if the patient is haemodynamically compromised.

Otherwise:
- Consider digoxin in an attempt to slow ventricular rate.

- Consider amiodarone.
- Consider heparinization, because there is growing evidence that the risk of systemic embolism is as significant with atrial flutter as it is with atrial fibrillation.

PAROXYSMAL ATRIAL TACHYCARDIA

- Adenosine has become the mainstay of treatment.
- If adenosine is unsuccessful, then consider verapamil (40–120 mg tds p.o.; alternatively 5–10 mg i.v. over 2–3 min), β-blockers (particularly the short-acting agent esmolol, 50–200 µg/kg/min by i.v. infusion), flecainide, sotalol or amiodarone.

In the patient with a tachydysrhythmia:
- Accurate haemodynamic assessment is the first priority.
- If there is no haemodynamic problem and the patient does not have chest pain, take time to think.
- Scrutinize the ECG as has been described.
- A broad-complex tachycardia is VT until proved otherwise: treatment for SVT when the rhythm is ventricular in origin is potentially disastrous for the patient.
- In atrial fibrillation, consider cardioversion (with electricity or with drugs) only if the patient is unstable haemodynamically or if you can be certain that the atria have been fibrillating for less than 48 h.
- Many antiarrhythmic drugs are negatively inotropic and in combination even more so. Avoid polypharmacy and be wary of the patient with impaired left ventricular function.

See *Cardiology*, Sections 1.1, 1.2 and 1.3.
1 Mayet J, More RS, Sutton GC. Anticoagulation for cardioversion of atrial dysrhythmias. *Eur Heart J* 1998; 19: 548–552.
2 West N. Broad complex tachycardia: assessment and management. CPD. *J Int Med* 1999; 1 (2): 50–56.
3 West N. Broad complex tachycardia. In: Davies C, Bashir Y, eds. *Cardiovascular Emergencies*. London: BMJ Books. Due to be published 2000.
4 Escoubet B, Coumel P, Poirier J-M *et al.* Suppression of dysrhythmias within hours after a single oral dose of amiodarone and relation to plasma and myocardial concentrations. *Am J Cardiol* 1985; 15: 696–702.

1.5 Nocturnal dyspnoea

Case history

A 70-year-old man has suffered recurrent episodes of nocturnal breathlessness for approximately 2 weeks. These episodes have woken him in the early hours and have become progressively more severe. You are called to see him as an emergency in the Medical Assessment Unit at 07.00 am one morning after he has suffered his worst episode of breathlessness to date.

Clinical approach

The differential diagnosis of recurrent nocturnal dyspnoea in an adult is not vast. Nevertheless, the two most likely pathologies, namely left ventricular failure and acute asthma, can be astonishingly difficult to distinguish from one another and, to make things challenging, prompt treatment is mandatory for each condition. In this case:
- Having ensured that the airway is safe, assess ventilation and circulation.
- Administer high-flow O_2.
- Obtain venous access.
- Measure arterial blood gases, paying attention to the parameters of acid–base balance as well as to those of gas exchange.
- Organize a chest radiograph.
- Do the cardiovascular signs and respiratory signs point convincingly to heart failure or to asthma?
- Consider immediate treatment measures, which may include diuretics, bronchodilators and steroids.

History of the presenting problem

This man may not be in a fit state to give a lengthy history, but can he give any details helpful in diagnosis? Ask about:
- History of previous heart trouble: myocardial infarction or angina?
- Has cardiac pain accompanied the episodes of dyspnoea?
  If he has either of these things, then left ventricular failure (LVF) is likely.

Note that:
- Dyspnoea is exacerbated by recumbency in both asthma and LVF, but a prompt and striking improvement on sitting upright is more likely in LVF.
- Cough on recumbency is a symptom of both conditions but cough and/or wheeze with typical diurnal variation outside of the acute attack is very suspicious of asthma.

Examination

Is the man well, ill, very ill or nearly dead? Can he speak in sentences? Is he cyanosed? Does he look exhausted? If he cannot speak, looks blue and tired—call for intensive care unit (ICU) help immediately. If he is not that bad, proceed with examination. Fear and hyperventilation are present equally in both asthma and pulmonary oedema.

Cardiovascular

Concentrate on the following:
- What is his heart rate and is he in sinus rhythm? Sinus tachycardia does not distinguish between asthma and heart failure. Although the presence of an abnormal rhythm does point towards a primary cardiovascular

problem, tachydysrhythmia can occasionally complicate asthma or its treatment.
- Check blood pressure, paradox and peripheral perfusion, but remember that the cardiovascular findings may be abnormal in acute asthma just as in LVF. However, the presence of paradox is suggestive of asthma if cardiac tamponade can be excluded.
- Where is the JVP? An elevated venous pressure is usually indicative of heart failure but this can be very difficult to identify in someone who is hyperventilating and frightened and can also be seen in acute asthma.
- Are there added heart sounds or murmurs? Their presence may suggest primary cardiac pathology although by themselves they do not secure the diagnosis.

Respiratory

The acute asthmatic typically breathes at high lung volumes and the person with heart failure often sounds bubbly. Pink bubbles frothing from the mouth secure the diagnosis of acute pulmonary oedema.

Asthma vs pulmonary oedema: some myths exploded!
- Generalized polyphonic wheezing is common in heart failure.
- Basal crackles are a completely non-specific sign of airway opening and will appear during a normal tidal inspiration if closing volume exceeds functional residual capacity.
- Acute pulmonary oedema may be completely silent with no wheezes or crackles on auscultation.

On examination, your patient has widespread wheezing as well as basal crackles. The venous pressure is elevated and he has a gallop rhythm with a third heart sound.

Approach to investigations and management

Investigations

Electrocardiogram

An ECG should be performed immediately in order to:
- Exclude an acute or previous myocardial infarct.
- Seek evidence of myocardial ischaemia.
- Assess the heart rhythm.

The ECG of your patient shows sinus tachycardia with a ventricular rate of 120 beats/min and has non-specific abnormalities of S-T/T segments in the lateral leads.

Chest radiograph

This may be the final arbiter between asthma and heart failure (Fig. 13).

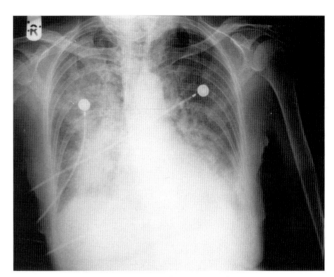
Fig. 13 Chest radiograph showing left ventricular failure.

Blood tests

Organize routine haematology, biochemistry and cardiac enzymes as well as arterial blood gases.

Echocardiography

Echocardiography is increasingly available as an emergency investigation and, in this situation, is particularly helpful in assessing left ventricular function. A normal left ventricle makes the diagnosis of heart failure untenable.

Management

Differentiating LVF from acute severe asthma can be difficult since many physical signs are common to both conditions. Do not spend hours agonizing over the differential diagnosis: action is called for.
- There is no harm in treating with nebulized bronchodilators in either condition.
- A bolus dose of corticosteroids will not harm someone in heart failure.
- It is better not to dehydrate the acute asthmatic, but intravenous diuretic should be administered given the exigencies of the situation. This is better than failing to treat heart failure promptly.
- Opiates can be of great benefit in heart failure, but you must be certain of the diagnosis.

Acute asthma + opiates = assisted ventilation or death.

Following emergency investigation and treatment, consider other possible diagnoses:
- Aspiration can present as nocturnal dyspnoea. Lying flat in bed at night predisposes to gastro-oesophageal

reflux and aspiration can be recurrent. Moreover, there is an association between acid in the lower oesophagus and bronchial hyperreactivity.
• PE causes acute dyspnoea, wheeze can be a prominent feature of its presentation and an elevated JVP is a common feature (see *Cardiology*, Section 1.9 and *Respiratory medicine*, Section 1.5).

You administer an intravenous bolus of 80 mg furosemide (frusemide) to your patient. He seems to improve a bit with this, and your diagnosis of LVF is confirmed by the typical appearances of pulmonary oedema on the chest radiograph. However, he remains breathless and is hypoxic with a PaO_2 of 8.5 kPa on 60% inspired O_2. What do you do now?

Acute pulmonary oedema not improving—what do you do?

This man is dangerously ill and might arrest soon. Call for help from the ICU:
• Give O_2 at 15 L/min through a mask with a reservoir bag. This should deliver 85% O_2.
• Give more intravenous furosemide; at least the same dose again.
• With a secure diagnosis of LVF, give a small dose (2.5–5 mg) of intravenous diamorphine.
• Consider attempting to reduce venous return with intravenous nitrates if blood pressure will allow.
• Consider elective ventilation.
Think further about the reason for his developing acute LVF:
• Are there any heart murmurs? Acute mitral regurgitation and ventricular septal defect are both complications of myocardial infarction (Fig. 14).
• Does a repeated ECG show evidence of evolving myocardial infarction?

• Could he have experienced a sudden nocturnal rise in blood pressure as is described with renovascular disease (see *Nephrology*, Sections 1.11 and 2.5.1) and developed pulmonary oedema as a result?
• Request an urgent echocardiogram.

 Are the heart rate and rhythm appropriate? In the case described, the heart rate and rhythm seem entirely appropriate for the clinical situation, but always consider that a primary dysrhythmia may be responsible for the heart failure, in which case its correction may be the most important therapeutic manoeuvre.

Further considerations if the patient still fails to respond

How much should you do?

If the measures described above are unsuccessful, should you proceed to more intensive treatment with insertion of a pulmonary arterial catheter, comprehensive haemodynamic monitoring and perhaps mechanical ventilation?

This difficult decision should be made by senior medical staff, with as complete a knowledge of the clinical situation as possible. It is vital to collect previous facts to build a clear picture of the patient's premorbid state. An echocardiograph 6 months previously which documented 'poor left ventricular function', together with a significantly compromised premorbid exercise tolerance would not augur well for a favourable outcome in intensive care. The considered views of the patient cannot sensibly be obtained when they are *in extremis*, but if they are known (living wills, etc.) then they should be considered (see *General clinical issues*, Section 3).

A decision not to intensify medical treatment should only be made for the reason that it would not benefit the

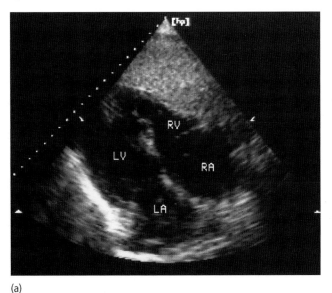
(a)

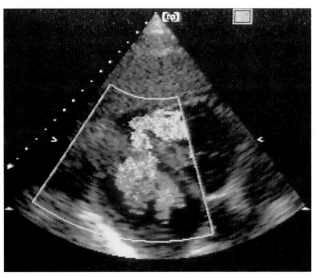
(b)

Fig. 14 (a) Echocardiogram of a ventricular septal defect following myocardial infarction; (b) shows flow across the defect.

patient. In this circumstance it is misleading and improper to speak in terms of 'denying' someone treatment. Anyone who has cared for a patient with a myocardium like a paper bag, who is ventilated mechanically and with cardiac output barely sustained on full inotropic support, appreciates that technology adds nothing to care in such cases and merely extends the agony of an inevitable outcome for all concerned.

Whilst efforts must be made to avoid this scenario, there often is not much information available in the receiving room when initial resuscitation fails. Protocols cannot be written for these situations, management decisions rest on individual assessment and obtaining senior help, but if in doubt the default position should be to treat whilst getting as much objective evidence as possible. In this example of intractable heart failure, for example, good-quality echocardiography would be very valuable in assessing cardiac function.

Ethical matters are discussed further in the case history that follows the description of a patient with an acute exacerbation of chronic airways obstruction (see Section 1.10, p. 37). It is vital that such considerations are discussed and that we debate and share them throughout our professional lives. It is unlikely, though, that hard and fast rules will ever be forthcoming and appropriate decision-making will continue to depend on obtaining the details of a patient's previous medical history, careful clinical assessment, objective measurements, experience of the doctor, and—let's not forget—medical common sense, defined by Richard Asher as the 'ability to see the obvious amidst confusion'.

 See *Cardiology*, Sections 1.6, 1.7 and 2.3 and associated references.

1.6 Bradydysrhythmia

Case history

A woman of 85 years has been found collapsed by a care assistant at her warden-controlled accommodation. She is normally quite active, mobile and self-caring but she does suffer occasional chest pain and takes antianginal medication in the form of regular oral nitrates.

It is 09.00 am when you are called to see her and the nursing staff are concerned that she has a pulse rate of 30 beats/min.

Clinical approach

Your immediate priorities are to:

• Resuscitate as necessary (airway, breathing, circulation) and get venous access.
• Organize an ECG—identify the heart rate and rhythm.
• Administer high-flow O$_2$ while arterial blood gases and acid–base balance are being measured.
• Measure blood pressure, assess cardiac output and conscious level. Look for evidence of heart failure and record other vital signs including temperature (probably measured rectally and with a low-reading thermometer if necessary).
• Comprehensive general and neurological examination follows if the patient is haemodynamically stable.

 Pulse 30 beats/min: the first priority is to assess the need for cardiovascular support, including treatment options aimed at normalizing heart rate.

History of the presenting problem

Obtain as much information as you can about this woman's acute illness. Can she give any sort of history? If not, when was she last seen by her neighbours or carers and was she in good health at that time? Is there any evidence that she may have spent the night on the floor of her bedroom? Has she been incontinent? Was she fully clothed when found and what was the ambient temperature of her surroundings? In addition:

• Enquire regarding her premorbid state of health: is there any specific history of medical or mental illness?
• Seek details of regular medication and enquire if any pills were found with her. Could she have taken an overdose—β-blockers, perhaps?

Examination

The cardiovascular findings are paramount but, if her condition is stable, concentrate on the following:

• Vital signs—what is her temperature?
• Pressure area: damage or bruising?
• Any findings that suggest hypothyroidism?

 Vital signs:
• Assess conscious level, recording your findings by means of the GCS. Is there anything to suggest that she has had a fit (tongue biting, incontinence)? Perform a careful neurological examination.
• Abnormal respiratory signs: aspiration or hypostatic pneumonia commonly complicates collapse in the elderly for whatever cause.
• Evidence of abdominal pathology: is there peritonism? This is easy to miss in this context if you do not look specifically.

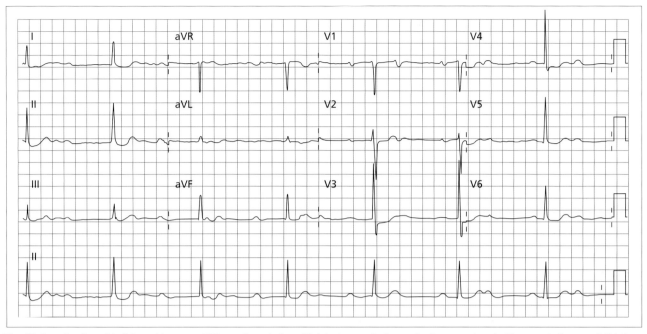

Fig. 15 Complete heart block but with narrow QRS complexes (a focus high in the ventricular conducting system) and with a ventricular rate of 41/min. This patient may not need immediate pacing; the decision will rest with the clinical situation. See text.

Approach to investigations and management

Investigations

An ECG will have been performed:
• Is there evidence of heart block and, if so, is it first-, second- or third-degree in type? (Fig. 15).
• Alternatively, there may be atrial fibrillation with a slow ventricular response or even profound sinus bradycardia.
• Is there indication of recent myocardial infarction which would demand specific treatment?

Generally speaking, the higher the degree of heart block, the less stable the situation. This, however, is by no means always the case and the decision to pace a patient should not be taken on the ECG alone (see below under Management).

In addition, check:
• Arterial blood: the presence of a metabolic acidosis is likely to indicate lactate accumulation as a result of compromised cardiac output.
• Routine haematology and biochemistry: in particular, request urgent electrolytes and renal function tests. You must ascertain that sodium and (especially) potassium levels are normal. If creatinine is raised, could this be acute renal failure from rhabdomyolysis? (see *Nephrology*, Section 1.17).
• Thyroid function tests: it is very difficult to diagnose thyroid imbalance in the elderly (see *Endocrinology*, Sections 1.14 and 2.3).
• Blood sugar: mandatory in all who have 'collapsed'.

• Chest radiograph: may reveal heart failure or pulmonary pathology.

Management of bradycardia

This is dictated by the clinical state of the patient.

The patient is well

Even a woman of 85 years may tolerate complete heart block at a pulse rate of 30 beats/min if her left ventricular function is good. She may be fully conscious with a normal blood pressure and warm peripheries. If this is the case, immediate transvenous pacing almost certainly is not necessary and an elective decision on the need for a permanent pacing system can be taken—unless there is a clear precipitant, e.g. β-blocker therapy, then she will certainly need one.

Close observation and cardiac monitoring is mandatory.

The patient is unwell

It is more likely that the patient will be hypotensive, cold, clammy and perhaps have a reduced conscious level. If this is the case, immediate temporary cardiac pacing is indicated.

Two other points should be made:
1 Marked bradydysrhythmia in someone who has suffered loss of consciousness, albeit transient, is almost certainly an indication for cardiac pacing, and the decision between a temporary, transvenous procedure (see Section 3, p. 97) or emergency insertion of a permanent system will depend upon local resources.

2 Heart block with normal, narrow QRS complexes (<120 ms), suggesting a nodal source of ventricular depolarization (Fig. 15), is less likely to require an immediate temporary pacemaker.

In the case described, the patient is shut down peripherally and has a systolic blood pressure of 80 mmHg. The ECG shows complete heart block with widened QRS complexes of 150 ms duration. The need for pacing is clear. But consider:
• Atropine (initial dose of 0.5–1 mg i.v.; further boluses can be given). This may speed ventricular rate and buy time while temporary pacing is organized.
• In extreme circumstances, an isoprenaline infusion may be used, again in an attempt to buy time (infusion rate, 2–10 μg/min, with drug half-life of approximately 2 min).
• The external cardiac pacemaker (see Section 3, p. 96) may be tried while arrangements are made for a definitive procedure. Sometimes, despite optimal application, the external system will not work. If this is the case, do not waste time agitating over it—isoprenaline and transvenous pacing will be the order of the day.

Management of specific causes of bradycardia

Myocardial infarction

The combination of acute myocardial infarction and bradydysrhythmia requiring temporary pacing presents an interesting challenge! The indications for acute pacing in this situation are straightforward enough, but the procedure obviously carries extra risk following thrombolysis.

Under these circumstances, attempt to insert the pacing wire through the femoral vein (the brachial is an alternative route but manoeuvring the tip of the wire is often very difficult) and then thrombolyse. If there is bleeding, then pressure can be exerted on these sites, whereas it is impossible in the neck. If these approaches prove impossible, insert the wire through the internal jugular or subclavian vein in the usual way—but most authorities would then advocate that thrombolysis should not be undertaken.

Some prefer to use tpa if a temporary pacing wire has been inserted, but there is no strong supporting evidence for this opinion.

 Consider the possibility of non-cardiac primary pathology in the bradyarrhythmic patient.

Hypothermia

A core body temperature of less than 33°C is diagnostic of hypothermia (Fig. 16). The management principles differ according to the cause of the lowered temperature.

RAPID ONSET

In the young, the lowering of body temperature is often rapid, e.g. after immersion in water or collapse on a cold city street with alcohol intoxication. Rapid ('active', 'intensive') warming is required: warm water immersion, warm peritoneal dialysis, etc.

GRADUAL ONSET

In most cases of hypothermia in the elderly, the fall in body temperature occurs over several days and warming should be more gentle (warm bedding, space blanket); indeed there is some evidence that intensive warming in the elderly causes cardiovascular collapse and dysrhythmias.

It is unlikely that the patient described here will be significantly hypothermic. Nevertheless, measure body temperature carefully: axillary temperatures are useless, oral measurement is notoriously badly performed and tympanic thermometers are not always available. Nurses are reluctant to measure rectal temperatures but sometimes they are essential and if hypothermia is a possibility then a low-reading thermometer must be used.

Steroids have been used in hypothermia but there is no documented evidence of their usefulness. It is reasonable to give intravenous methylprednisolone (40–100 mg) in extreme cases on the basis that there is nothing to lose if the core temperature is less than 29°C and conscious level is impaired.

In the acute situation with a cold, semiconscious patient, broad-spectrum antibiotics should be given empirically: pneumonia (both hypostatic and aspiration) is a complicating feature of abnormally low body temperature.

Hypothyroidism

Hypothyroidism is associated with a variety of bradydysrhythmias, particularly sinus bradycardia and atrial fibrillation with a slow ventricular rate.

Extreme presentation of hypothyroidism is rare and tends to be the preserve of the elderly. If thyroid function is severely deficient in the acute setting, then steroids are life-saving and should be administered before replacement of thyroid hormone. Without them, thyroid replacement therapy can result in acute circulatory collapse.

Care is required in the prescription of thyroid hormone. It should be presumed that elderly patients will have coexisting ischaemic heart disease and that hypothyroidism will have developed over a considerable period of time. Vigorous replacement of thyroid hormone may

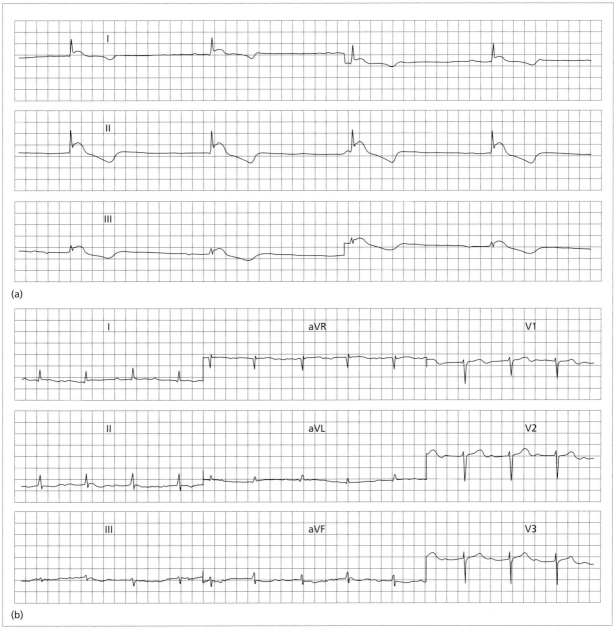

Fig. 16 This patient had a core temperature of 25°C on admission. (a) The first ECG shows sinus bradycardia, first-degree heart block and prominent 'J' waves. (b) The second trace shows the pattern at 31°C: first-degree heart block, rate of 75/min and no 'J' waves.

well do more harm than good. Hence the starting dose of thyroxine should be very small, 25 µg daily or even on alternate days.

Triiodothyronine is rarely indicated: it should be given only in extreme cases, and then cautiously.

Bradycardia is a challenging problem:
- Be clear regarding the priorities, and support the cardiovascular system before all else.
- Understand the indications for cardiac pacing.
- Do not just think about the heart: could there be a non-cardiological reason for the bradydysrhythmia?

See *Cardiology*, Sections 1.3 and 2.2.1; *Endocrinology*, Sections 1.14 and 2.3; *Medicine for the elderly*, Section 2.5.

1.7 Acute severe asthma

Case history

A 48-year-old woman who has had asthma for 10 years is admitted to the A&E by her general practitioner with an exacerbation of wheezy dyspnoea. On arrival she is cyanosed and unable to speak.

Clinical approach

Resuscitation is the first priority. Cyanosis in acute asthma is an ominous finding: when it is detectable clinically the PaO_2 is likely to be less than 6 kPa.

Administer:

• Maximum inspired O_2 by face mask. This is best achieved by using a mask with a reservoir bag that can deliver inspired O_2 concentrations of 85% at a flow rate of 15 L/min. Do not be concerned about high-flow O_2 in this situation: it will not cause progressive hypoventilation and hypercapnia, although these might occur if the patient gets exhausted.

• Nebulized bronchodilators. Salbutamol 5–10 mg should be mixed with ipatropium bromide (Atrovent 500 µg) in a nebulizer chamber and the patient should receive the drugs as soon as possible, ensuring that the nebulizer is driven by O_2 (see below under Management hazard).

Ensure:

• Venous access: two large peripheral veins should be cannulated immediately. Use grey venflons in the antecubital fossae if at all possible. If a peripheral line cannot be achieved, then insert a femoral line. Avoid subclavian or internal jugular cannulation—an iatrogenic pneumothorax is not a good idea, and line insertion will interfere with important resuscitation procedures at the head end of the patient.

Give:

• Steroids, 30–60 mg prednisolone orally (or 200 mg hydrocortisone intravenously if there is any concern regarding absorption by the oral route).

• An infusion of intravenous bronchodilator in severe cases (see below).

Measure:

• Highest priority—arterial blood gases.

• A base-line peak expired flow rate (PEFR) or forced expired volume in 1 second (FEV_1) if possible—but these measurements may well be impractical in the distressed and dyspnoeic asthmatic.

Bad asthma—oximetry gives only part of the picture:
• Oximetry quantifies arterial oxygenation but does not tell you how well a patient is ventilating: a patient given high-flow O_2 might not be hypoxic but could still be hypoventilating, significantly hypercapnic and at risk of respiratory arrest.
• The usual cause of hypoxia in acute asthma is a ventilation/perfusion defect: unless there is an obligatory shunt, e.g. due to complicating lobar or segmental lung collapse, the hypoxia of acute asthma will be corrected by high-flow O_2.
• Blood gases provide information on acid–base balance. A metabolic acidosis in acute asthma is a bad prognostic sign, suggesting impaired cardiac output due to the severe airflow obstruction. Oximetry provides no clue in this direction.

Asthmatics are not always breathless due to asthma. Consider other causes of acute, 'noisy' dyspnoea and potential complications of asthma:
• Upper airway obstruction—this can mimic an exacerbation of asthma and might be caused by anaphylaxis, epiglottitis, severe tracheitis or a foreign body.
• Spontaneous pneumothorax—a recognized complication of acute severe asthma.

Both of these events are life threatening and require immediate treatment.

History of presenting problem

An acute exacerbation of asthma usually develops over several days and the symptoms commonly show diurnal variation with nocturnal distress being prominent. It is not always possible to identify a precipitating cause but unusual allergenic exposure (contact with animals, moving into a new house, cleaning carpets, a seasonal factor, e.g. grass or tree pollen) and viral upper respiratory tract infections are common culprits and the relevant history should be sought.

Consider alternative diagnoses in the wheezy, dyspnoeic patient:

• Stridor can be mistaken for wheeze—is large airway obstruction a possibility?

• Wheezing can be a prominent feature of LVF (see Section 1.5, p. 19).

• Wheezing is an occasional presenting symptom of PE (see Section 1.8, p. 28).

Relevant past history

It is helpful to know how troublesome the patient's asthma was before the acute attack since previous history is helpful in predicting outcome [1]. If the patient can give an account, then ask:

• How long have symptoms been deteriorating before the current presentation?

• How frequent have acute exacerbations been in the past?

• How good was asthma control before the exacerbation began?

• How long had symptoms been deteriorating before admission to hospital?

• What regular medication does she use for asthma control?

These features may indicate how difficult the underlying condition is to treat. Knowledge of the severity of previous acute attacks is also important. Has she ever been admitted to hospital before with an acute attack? Has she ever needed ventilation? In an individual asthmatic patient, recurrent attacks tend to be similar, both in severity and in speed of recovery.

If background control has been poor, recovery following treatment is often delayed, as it is when symptoms

Table 6 Clinical signs which correlate with the severity of acute asthma.

Inability to speak
Cyanosis
Use of accessory muscles of ventilation and a hyperinflated chest
Reduced tidal volume, the extreme example being the silent chest
Pulsus paradoxus; there is a correlation between degree of paradox and severity of airways' obstruction
Measurement of PEFR or FEV₁ is often impossible in the acute attack but should be carried out as soon as practicable. This will provide a base-line for future recovery

FEV_1, forced expired volume in 1 s; PEFR, peak expired flow rate.

have been deteriorating for a week or more prior to admission. Late-onset asthma (as suffered, by definition, by the patient described here) is often more difficult to manage, both acutely and chronically, than early-onset asthma.

 In the bad asthmatic—as in many other things—to be forewarned is to be forearmed.

Examination

Is the patient well, ill, very ill or nearly dead? If the latter—call the ICU for help immediately.

Careful cardiorespiratory examination is mandatory. Be aware of those physical signs that correlate with severity of the acute attack of asthma (Table 6).

Note also the following, and do not be misled.

Respiratory rate

It is important to measure respiratory rate, but the degree of tachypnoea does not correlate with the severity of an asthma attack. Asthma is a terrifying condition and the vast majority of acute asthmatics hyperventilate, but respiratory rate falls as the asthmatic becomes exhausted with the effort of breathing—eventually leading to hypercapnic respiratory failure and the need for ventilatory support. Does the patient look exhausted?

- An acute attack of asthma causes hyperventilation.
- At the moment of death the respiratory rate is zero.
- A normal respiratory rate does not necessarily mean that the patient is 'fine'.

Wheeze on auscultation

Widespread wheezing indicates marked airways obstruction, but beware the asthmatic who has a silent chest on auscultation. Tidal volume may be reduced so much by airways obstruction that insufficient flow is being generated to create wheeze.

Cardiovascular signs

Sinus tachycardia is common in acute asthma and does not correlate with severity. Fear, increased sympathetic drive and bronchodilator drugs all contribute to a rise in pulse rate and bradycardia may supervene as hypoxia becomes more marked.

The degree of pulsus paradoxus does correlate with severity as it reflects the abnormal changes in transpulmonary pressure generated by increasing airways obstruction.

 Examination of the bad asthmatic:
- Exclude pneumothorax—a life-threatening complication of asthma.
- Differentiate stridor from wheeze—a life-threatening alternative diagnosis.

 Bad asthma:
- No clinical sign correlates well with the degree of hypoxia, emphasizing the need to measure arterial blood gases at the earliest opportunity.

Approach to investigations and management

Investigations

How severe is the attack?

Check arterial blood gases and measure airways obstruction, as detailed above.

Chest radiograph

This should be taken (and looked at!) as soon as possible:
- Exclude pneumothorax.
- Is there an area of consolidation, perhaps due to superadded infection?
- Is there segmental collapse due to sputum plugging?

Blood tests

Note the following:
- Full blood count: anaemia will compound impaired tissue O_2 delivery in a patient who is likely to be hypoxaemic.
- Electrolytes: β_2-agonists, theophyllines and steroids all predispose to hypokalaemia, which creates a respiratory myopathy. The acute asthmatic needs his respiratory pump!

 Blood gases in asthma:
Ask advice from the ICU regarding any patient with:
- A Pa_{CO_2} above 5 kPa—a normal or elevated Pa_{CO_2} indicates failing respiratory effort.
- A base deficit of >10 mmol/L—metabolic acidosis indicates compromised cardiac output.

Management

Oxygen and fluids

Sufficient O_2 should be given to correct hypoxia.

Hyperventilation and poor oral intake can lead to dehydration and this is to be avoided:
• Dry bronchial secretions are more difficult to clear and are more likely to lead to sputum plugging.
• A relatively high right ventricular filling pressure is necessary in severe airways obstruction in order to safeguard cardiac output.
• Do not be frightened to give intravenous crystalloid: 1 L in the first 1–2 h is entirely reasonable.
• Correct hypokalaemia vigorously if this is present.

Nebulized bronchodilators

These should be used routinely. There is evidence that combining anticholinergic drugs with β_2-agonists confers additional benefit in acute asthma [2,3]. Nebulized therapy should be repeated frequently in the early stages of the acute attack: salbutamol (5–10 mg) can be mixed and nebulized with ipratropium (500 μg) and repeated after 30 min if necessary.

Continuous nebulization is an alternative approach which is used more commonly in the United States.

Intravenous bronchodilators

Intravenous, as well as nebulized, bronchodilators should be administered to severe asthmatics, such as the patient described here. It is better to overtreat at first and then to withdraw the intravenous infusion than to be several steps behind with medication as you struggle to keep the patient off a ventilator. Consider several things when you choose intravenous medication:
• Use aminophylline with caution—it is possible to push someone into toxic levels with intravenous aminophylline if oral theophyllines are part of their regular medication. The potential complications of aminophylline toxicity—epileptic convulsions and/or vomiting—are extremely dangerous in acute asthma [4].
• Salbutamol is the alternative and is preferred by many—dilute 5 mg in 500 mL 5% dextrose or 0.9% saline and start infusion at a rate of 7.5 μg/min, titrating according to response. The main side effects are tachycardia and tremor.

β_2-Agonists and aminophylline must always be given with O_2, not instead of it.
These drugs are pulmonary vasodilators as well as bronchodilators and their administration can rapidly worsen the ventilation/perfusion mismatch which is the cause of hypoxia in asthma. They can therefore cause reduction in arterial O_2 tension unless supplemental O_2 is given.

Steroids

Give prednisolone (30–60 mg) orally if possible.

There is no evidence that hydrocortisone confers additional benefit in acute asthma but, in the severely ill patient, intravenous corticosteroids should be given to obviate problems of absorption. Under these circumstances hydrocortisone (200 mg) can be given over 5–10 min.

Assessing recovery

As well as careful clinical appraisal at regular intervals:
• Airways obstruction should be monitored frequently using either PEFR or FEV_1.
• Repeat arterial blood gases if arterial O_2 saturation is <92% or if hypercapnia or metabolic acidosis has been recorded on the previous measurement.

In acute severe asthma, regular reassessment during the first hours of recovery is essential. This must include:
• clinical reappraisal
• measurement of airways obstruction
• repeat blood gas estimation as indicated.
Remember:
• always seek early senior review
• if the patient does not improve and assisted ventilation becomes necessary, the move to the ICU should be by cool elective decision, not in a panic when the patient is close to respiratory arrest.

See *Respiratory medicine*, Sections 1.1, 1.7, 1.14 and 2.2.2.
Ali NJ. Acute severe asthma: assessment and treatment. CPD *J Int Med* 1999; 1(1): 9–12.
1 Jenkins PF, Benfield GFA, Smith AP. Predicting recovery from acute severe asthma. *Thorax* 1981; 36: 835–841.
2 Rebuck AS, Chapman KS, Arbound R *et al.* Nebulized anticholinergic and sympathomimetic treatment of asthma and chronic bronchitis in the emergency room. *Am J Med* 1987; 82: 59–64.
3 O'Driscoll BR, Taylor RJ, Horsley MG *et al.* Nebulized salbutamol with and without ipratropium bromide in acute airflow obstruction. *Lancet* 1989; ii: 1418–1420.
4 Huang D, O'Brien RG, Harman E *et al.* Does aminophylline benefit adults admitted to the hospital for acute exacerbation of asthma? *Ann Intern Med* 1993; 119: 1155–1160.

1.8 Pleurisy

Case history

A 22-year-old woman, Miss G, is referred to the A&E by her general practitioner because of sudden onset of right-sided, pleuritic chest pain. She has no previous medical or surgical history. She works in one of the local High Street banks where she is engaged to be married to one of the deputy managers. She has taken oral contraception for the past 12 months. When you see her, she is in some pain but her vital signs are normal.

Clinical approach

There are no prizes for making the diagnosis! This is PE until proved otherwise. Your priorities are described below.

Resuscitation

• Assess airway, breathing, circulation.
• Cardiovascular collapse would mean major PE and be an indication for thrombolysis.
• High-flow O_2 should be administered unless hypoxia is excluded by normal pulse oximetry or arterial blood gases on air.
• Obtain venous access and administer intravenous fluid if the patient is hypotensive.

Heparinize

Heparin should be administered without delay to protect against further embolization. Doctors often delay giving heparin until they have completed taking the history, examining the patient and obtaining the result of initial investigations. Why? If it is clear that PE is the number one diagnosis—start treatment.

Analgesia

Pleurisy is (by definition) painful: relieve the pain as soon as possible, apart from anything else a patient who is comfortable can provide a much clearer (and quicker) history than one who is finding it hard to take a breath, let alone answer questions.

 NSAIDs are excellent for relieving the pain of pleurisy, but opiates may be required as well.

Immediate assessment

Miss G has normal cardiovascular findings. Her PaO_2 on air is 11.5 kPa, $PaCO_2$ is 3 kPa and her standard base excess is –1. Her pain is improved considerably with a Voltarol suppository, you have good venous access and she has received a subcutaneous dose of low-molecular-weight heparin. In other words, there are no immediately worrying features and anticoagulation has been commenced. Proceed with clinical assessment as follows.

History of presenting problem

Enquire about the following salient points:

• Has the patient ever had anything like this before? What diagnosis (if any) was made?
• Did the pain start suddenly or gradually? The former is typical of PE, but a gradual onset of symptoms does not exclude the diagnosis.
• Sudden onset of pain (and/or breathlessness) after defaecation is highly suggestive of PE and there is commonly a story of becoming suddenly very frightened, '… something awful had happened, Doctor'. Ask specifically for these details if they are not volunteered.
• Predisposing factors for PE—oestrogen-containing contraceptives, pregnancy, recent surgery, immobility or long-distance travel are the obvious ones—but do not discount the diagnosis if there is no obvious precipitating cause: many people suffer PE for no apparent reason.
• Breathlessness—autopsy studies show that patients who die of PE virtually always have evidence that PEs have been going on for some time: has this patient, presenting with chest pain, had any problem breathing recently? Has she had to slow down over the last week or two?
• Haemoptysis—the commonest differential diagnosis of pleuritic chest pain due to PE is musculoskeletal pain, which does not cause haemoptysis.
• Calf/leg swelling or pain—these would suggest deep venous thrombosis (DVT) and enormously increase the probability that someone presenting with pleurisy had PE.
• Has anyone in the family had PE?

Although this patient has presented with pleurisy, always consider the diagnosis of PE in someone who presents with unexplained breathlessness (of sudden onset or otherwise). Suspicion will be heightened if the chest radiograph is normal. See *Respiratory medicine*, Section 1.1.

 Pitfalls in the diagnosis of PE

• Pleuritic pain is not always a feature of PE. With large, central emboli, cardiovascular collapse and/or breathlessness are much more common findings; it is the smaller, more peripheral embolus which tends to cause pain.
• The presenting history (and findings) may be dominated by secondary cardiac features—ischaemic cardiac pain and ECG changes. A PE creates a sudden increase in afterload on the right ventricle and resultant myocardial ischaemia may be a prominent feature of the history: 'secondary cardiac pain'. Moreover, if there is coronary artery disease with particular involvement of the left ventricle, the ECG may well show abnormalities which are left sided.

 PE—treat if in doubt!

Pulmonary embolic disease carries a significant mortality, the presenting features may be far from typical and predisposing factors for venous thrombosis are often not apparent.

Always have a high index of suspicion for this diagnosis and be prepared to anticoagulate empirically pending further investigations.

Differential diagnosis of pleurisy

The case described leaves little room for doubt, but always consider the following alternative diagnoses and take the history and perform your examination with these in mind:

- Spontaneous pneumothorax—heparin can convert this into a haemothorax!
- Pneumonia—fever is often a prominent symptom, and chest signs and radiography will usually show consolidation. Beware though: fever and radiographic consolidation can be a feature of pulmonary infarction.
- Musculoskeletal pain—this can be difficult to differentiate: the presence of chest wall tenderness does not necessarily distinguish it from pleurisy (particularly embolic pleurisy) and, if the diagnosis is unclear, anticoagulate until PE is excluded.
- Rare conditions—pleurisy can be the presenting symptom of systemic lupus erythematosus. Check relevant serology (antinuclear factor and DNA binding) and be particularly suspicious if pleurisy is recurrent.

Examination

The most important aspects are obviously cardiovascular and respiratory examination.

Cardiovascular

What does the patient look like? This patient seems pretty well, but check peripheral perfusion, pulse, blood pressure and JVP.

Look carefully for signs of pulmonary hypertension, which would strongly support the diagnosis of PE:
- Elevated venous pressure, particularly with an exaggerated 'a' wave.
- Right ventricular heave—which can develop surprisingly rapidly following an acute rise in pulmonary artery pressure.
- Loud pulmonary second sound.

Respiratory

A pleural rub may be present (though commonly is not) and it can be very evanescent. Always believe other medical staff if they describe a rub which is no longer present when you examine the patient.

Pleurisy can be associated with local chest wall tenderness. Patients will tell you that it has been uncomfortable lying on the affected side and they may be locally tender on palpation. This is an important point because local tenderness does not necessarily mean pain of musculoskeletal origin—another classic diagnostic 'catch'.

Other aspects

Search for a DVT, but do not be surprised if you do not find one and do not, whatever you do, let its absence put you off making the diagnosis of PE.

A rectal examination (and pelvic examination in women) will be necessary at some stage.

Approach to investigations and management

Investigations

Chest radiograph

An early chest radiograph is vital. In PE, the findings are usually normal but a number of radiographic abnormalities are described [1], including:
- line shadows at the bases
- peripheral wedge-shaped shadow(s)
- areas of relative oligaemia in the lung fields (rare)
- enlarged proximal pulmonary artery (rare).

Electrocardiogram

The ECG is commonly normal but it may show:
- T-wave inversion in V1–V3
- 'S1,Q3,T3' pattern—described in all the books and reflecting axis change as a result of a sudden increase in right ventricular afterload (Fig. 17)
- right atrial hypertrophy with a 'P pulmonale'
- right bundle branch block (can be normal variant, but significant if new)
- evidence of ischaemic change—which may be left or right sided (as discussed).

Blood gases

Blood gases typically show hypocapnia because of hyperventilation. Hypoxia may or may not be present. If there is a base deficit, your concerns should be heightened because it indicates secondary cardiovascular compromise.

Rapid definitive investigations

Ventilation/perfusion isotope lung scan is the commonest, readily available imaging test (Fig. 18) but CT angiography of the chest is increasingly used (Fig. 19). This technique is particularly valuable in those with chronic lung disease, the presence of which makes interpretation of ventilation/perfusion scans very difficult, and in confirming the anatomical extent of an embolus, which is important information before thrombolytic therapy is administered [2].

Other tests

Routine haematology and biochemical tests should be performed. Are there any clues to a systemic disease that might predispose to PE?

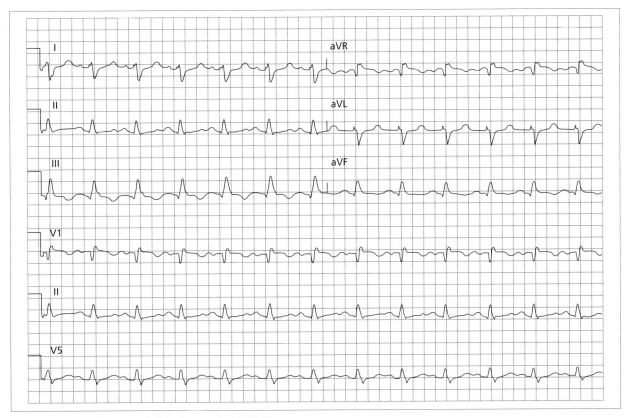

Fig. 17 ECG in acute pulmonary embolism showing the S1, Q3, T3 pattern.

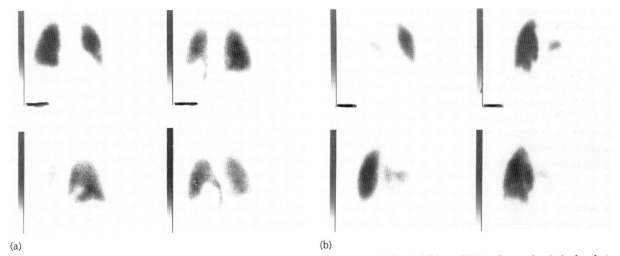

(a)   (b)

Fig. 18 Pulmonary emboli revealed on perfusion isotope lung scanning. (a) Large, segmental defect in left lung. (b) Virtually complete lack of perfusion in right lung. Ventilation scanning was normal in both patients.

Note that it is not possible to interpret the results of a thrombophilia screen in the presence of thrombus or anticoagulation.

Management

Anticoagulation or thrombolysis?

Heparin followed by warfarin will be appropriate for the majority of patients but, occasionally, thrombolytic agents will be indicated. This is a decision that should be taken at a senior level. There is no trial evidence to guide this decision, but a common view would be that thrombolysis is indicated in those patients who suffer persistent haemodynamic consequences from embolic disease despite heparin therapy.

The hypotensive, clammy patient

If there is significant haemodynamic disturbance then a high venous filling pressure is required to assist the struggling right ventricle. Give intravenous plasma expander (500 mL) and reassess. Detailed haemodynamic monitoring is ideal and these patients should be managed in an ICU.

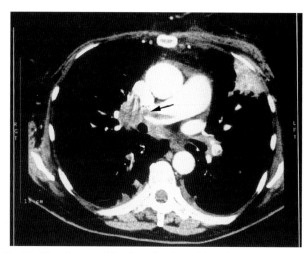

Fig. 19 CT angiogram of the chest showing a clot in the proximal pulmonary artery (arrowed).

Emboli despite anticoagulation

Repeated embolic events despite adequate anticoagulation may require mechanical intervention, e.g. insertion of a filter device into the inferior vena cava.

Pulmonary embolism

- PE is a common and potentially life-threatening condition.
- The presentation is often atypical. If confronted with unexplained breathlessness or collapse, question the possibility of PE. Large central emboli tend not to cause pain. Do not necessarily expect to find a predisposing cause for venous thrombosis. Always have a high index of suspicion.
- Examination is commonly unremarkable.
- The chest radiograph and ECG are commonly normal.
- Correct hypoxia and search critically for haemodynamic abnormalities.
- Ventilation/perfusion scans and CT angiography are particularly valuable soon after the clinical event: normal images obtained more than 48 h after the clinical event do not exclude PE.
- Anticoagulate promptly while investigations are organized and the diagnosis is clarified. Give heparin. If the patient is very ill, do not hesitate to seek senior advice—the next PE may be fatal—and consider thrombolysis.

See *Cardiology*, Section 1.9; *Respiratory medicine*, Section 1.5; *Haematology*, Sections 1.13, 1.20 and 3.6.

The PIOPED Investigation. Value of the ventilation/perfusion scan in acute pulmonary embolism: results of the prospective investigation of pulmonary embolism diagnosis. *JAMA* 1990; 263: 2753–2759.

Stein PD, Henry PW. Prevalence of acute pulmonary embolism in a general hospital and at autopsy. *Chest* 1995; 108: 4, 978–981.

Suspected acute pulmonary embolism: a practical approach. British Thoracic Society Standards of Care Committee. October 1997, Vol. 52, supplement 4.

1 Pulmonary thromboembolism. In: Fraser RS, Pare PD, eds. *Diagnosis of Diseases of the Chest*, 4d edn. Philadelphia: WB Saunders, 1999.

2 van Rossum AB, Treurniet FEE, Kieft GJ, Smith SJ, Schepers-Bok R. Role of spiral volumetric computed tomographic scanning in the assessment of patients with suspicion of pulmonary embolism and an abnormal ventilation/perfusion scan. *Thorax* 1996; 51: 23–28.

1.9 Community-acquired pneumonia

Case history

A 24-year-old man who is an accomplished rugby footballer and normally very fit, has been unwell for 12 h and his girlfriend has brought him to A&E on a Sunday morning where you are called to see him.

He describes feeling very cold while in the club-house bar after his rugby match on the preceding afternoon, after which he suffered a violent shaking attack. He went home and took himself off to bed where he felt extremely hot before falling asleep. He awoke 3 h later with right-sided lower lateral chest pain which was worse on inspiration. Pain persisted throughout the night and this, together with alternating episodes of feeling 'hot and cold' associated with rigors, resulted in a miserable night's sleep.

Clinical approach

Rapid onset of pyrexial illness with early appearance of pleuritic pain and rigors is a classical presentation of pneumococcal pneumonia. The first question to be asked is 'how ill is the patient?'—well, ill, very ill or nearly dead? If he is nearly dead, call the ICU immediately.

In this setting, one should be particularly concerned about:
- toxicity—i.e. high fever with or without the cardiovascular changes of sepsis
- confusion—a marker of severe illness due to hypoxia and/or sepsis.

Action

The priorities are:
- Give high-flow O_2, cannulate a large vein and infuse intravenous crystalloids.
- Take blood cultures and commence antibiotics: there is no place for delaying antibiotic therapy while you wait for a chest radiograph and a white cell count.
- For community-acquired pneumonia:
  - In the moderately sick patient, start with amoxycillin and a macrolide.
  - In the more severely ill patient, substitute a third-order cephalosporin for the penicillin and combine this with a macrolide.

• Immediate oximetry is mandatory. In anyone who is severely ill, or whenever O_2 saturation is <92%, arterial blood should be taken for blood gas analysis. This will provide information on oxygenation, ventilatory function (through $PaCO_2$) and acid–base balance.
• Urgent chest radiograph.

Severe pneumonia

If faced with a patient who is toxic, haemodynamically compromised, hypoxic or confused, consider the need for management on the ICU.

Ask this question early and continue to ask it as you assess progress following treatment: an elective decision to move the patient to the ICU is preferable to a mad rush down the hospital corridor in the early hours of the morning.

History of the presenting problem

There can be little doubt that this patient has community-acquired pneumonia. Some details in the history can help to identify the causative organism:
• Non-bacterial causes of pneumonia, e.g. *Mycoplasma pneumoniae*, are often characterized by a relatively long prodromal stage with severe general symptoms and only mild respiratory tract manifestations, especially in the first few days.
• Pleurisy is more common in bacterial than in non-bacterial pneumonia.
• Mental confusion is often prominent in *Legionella* pneumonia.
• Has the patient had 'flu?—staphylococcal pneumonia is a feared complication.

Examination

Aside from vital signs—temperature, pulse rate, respiratory rate and blood pressure—the two main issues to resolve are 'how ill is the patient'? and 'what are the chest signs'?

How ill is the patient?

The following suggest that the patient is very ill:
• difficulty in speaking
• patient looks exhausted
• use of accessory muscles
• cool peripheries
• cyanosis
• hypotension.

Respiratory

Check respiratory rate—remembering that tachypnoea is expected and that a normal respiratory rate may indicate exhaustion and be a very worrying finding. Listen for a pleural rub and signs of consolidation. In non-bacterial pneumonia the respiratory signs are commonly unimpressive; a pleural rub suggests bacterial pneumonia.

Approach to investigations and management

Investigations

Immediate oximetry is mandatory. In anyone who is severely ill, or whenever O_2 saturation is <95%, arterial blood should be taken for blood gas analysis. Rising $PaCO_2$ indicates failing ventilation and acidosis failing circulation: get ICU help if either are present.

Chest radiograph

'Milk' as much information as possible from the chest radiograph:
• Pneumococcal pneumonia presents classically as lobar or segmental consolidation (Fig. 20). Multiple, non-contiguous and sometimes bilateral segments may be affected.
• A variety of radiographic patterns are described in *Mycoplasma* pneumonia (Fig. 21) and in Legionnaires' disease [1,2].

In A&E, basic radiographic observations are more valuable than recognizing esoteric appearances:
• The worse the radiograph, the more you worry about the patient.
• Radiograph changes are not static; the radiograph may deteriorate during the early stage of treatment and in pneumococcal pneumonia the radiograph may be normal at presentation (even in the presence of a classical history and signs of consolidation on examination) only to become abnormal over the next few hours.

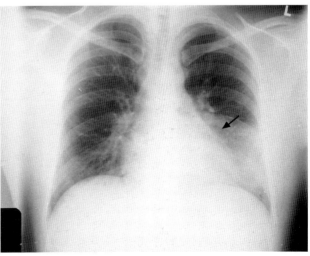

Fig. 20 Lingular consolidation due to *Pneumococcus*; the arrow marks an air bronchogram.

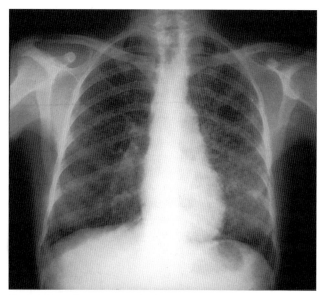

Fig. 21 *Mycoplasma* pneumonia, showing an unusual, lobular pattern of consolidation.

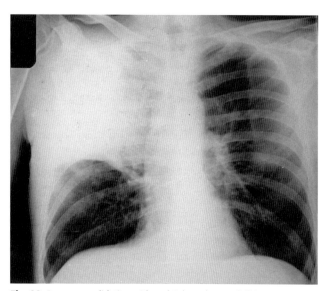

Fig. 22 Dense consolidation with no 'air bronchogram'. This was staphylococcal pneumonia following 'flu'.

• If the radiograph deteriorates despite antibiotic therapy, you may not be covering the correct organism or the diagnosis of infection may be incorrect. Consider other pathologies, such as pulmonary infarction, pulmonary eosinophilia, cryptogenic organizing pneumonia or pulmonary vasculitis (see *Respiratory medicine*, Sections 2.7.2, 2.8.3 and 2.8.4).
• The absence of an 'air bronchogram' within an area of consolidation suggests exudate or pus filling the conducting airways; organisms commonly responsible for this appearance are *Pneumococcus*, *Staphylococcus* (Fig. 22) and Gram-negatives. Also consider aspiration pneumonia or proximal bronchial obstruction, e.g. due to carcinoma or a foreign body.
• The presence of pleural fluid is suggestive of bacterial aetiology and, if there is a significant effusion, a diagnostic tap should be considered.

• Early cavitation in an area of consolidation is typical of staphylococcal infection, but consider Gram-negatives such as *Klebsiella* and do not forget tuberculosis.

Other tests

Check full blood count, electrolytes, and renal and liver function. Take blood for culture (and sputum if available). Take serum samples for serological testing and urine for assays of specific antigens. Remember the following:
• The patient with overwhelming sepsis may have a normal white cell count.
• The white cell count is a poor discriminator between bacterial and non-bacterial pneumonia.
• Uraemia is said to be a bad prognostic sign in pneumonia [3]. This is unlikely to be an abnormality specific to pneumonia, but more a general indicator of severity of illness when dehydration and catabolism both contribute to a rise in serum urea.
• Hyponatraemia is another non-specific indicator of severity of illness, although it may be a particular feature of Legionnaires' disease.

Management

Give O_2, high flow if necessary, to get PO_2 >92%.

Antibiotics

Antibiotics should be given without delay. The choice of antibiotics is guided by a knowledge of the pathogens that are most commonly implicated in community-acquired pneumonia—*Pneumococcus*, *Haemophilus* and some of the non-bacterial organisms.
• In the moderately sick patient, start with amoxycillin and a macrolide.
• In the more severely ill, substitute a third-order cephalosporin for the penicillin and combine this with a macrolide.
• If there is any suggestion of preceding influenza or a 'flu epidemic is in progress, add in a specific antistaphylococcal antibiotic, e.g. flucloxacillin.
• If Gram-negative infection or aspiration is suspected, modify your antibiotics appropriately.
• The patient with chronic respiratory disease will have additional management needs (see *Infectious diseases*, Section 1.4).

Give antibiotics intravenously to start with if the patient is moderately or severely unwell.

Fluids

Correct dehydration vigorously; hypovolaemia is a bad prognostic indicator in pneumonia.

Review

Plan to assess the response to treatment regularly, looking at:
- what does the patient look and feel like?
- clinical features—temperature, haemodynamics, respiratory rate
- physiological measures—oximetry and blood gases
- radiographic appearances.

If things are getting worse, not better, then call for help—elective intubation and ventilation are far preferable to 'crash calls'.

 Community-acquired pneumonia is a common medical emergency:
- Prompt clinical, radiographic and physiological assessment is the management priority.
- Early antibiotic therapy and vigorous fluid replacement are mandatory.
- The antibiotic combination will need to be modified if particular infections are suspected or in particular circumstances, e.g. immunosuppression.
- There should be a strategy for reviewing response to treatment.

 See *Infectious diseases*, Sections 1.2 and 1.4; *Respiratory medicine*, Section 1.10.

1 Jenkins PF, Miller AC, Osman J, Pearson SB, Rowley JM. Legionnaires disease; a clinical description of 13 cases. *Br J Dis Chest* 1979; 73: 31.
2 British Thoracic Society. British Thoracic Society guidelines on pneumonia. *Br J Hosp Med* 1993; 49(5): 346–350. (An update is due to be published in late 2000.)
3 Ali N, Andrews BE, Harrison BDW, Jenkins PF, Sillis M. Clinical spectrum and diagnosis of mycoplasma pneumoniae infection. *Q J Med* 1986; 58: 241–253.

1.10 Chronic airways obstruction

Case history

A 69-year-old man is admitted from his home with a history of cough and dyspnoea, both symptoms deteriorating for approximately 10 days. He is a regular attender at the local chest clinic where a diagnosis of chronic airways obstruction has been made; the old records have been found and delivered to the A&E where you assess the patient. He has smoked 20 cigarettes per day for 50 years.

Clinical approach

Your management priorities are:
- Resuscitate if necessary—assess airway, breathing and circulation.

- Obtain venous access and take arterial blood for blood gas analysis.
- Request an immediate chest radiograph.
- Administer O_2, the concentration delivered (FiO_2) depending on whether he is retaining CO_2 (see below under Management).
- Attempt a base-line measurement of the degree of airways obstruction with a PEFR or FEV_1. This may be impossible if the patient is breathless or otherwise distressed.
- Give nebulized bronchodilators, probably combining a β_2-agonist (5–10 mg salbutamol) with an anticholinergic (500 μg ipratropium bromide).
- If he is distressed or in pain, relieve symptoms but avoid the use of respiratory depressants if at all possible.
- Assess fluid balance and, if there is any suggestion of fluid overload, administer furosemide (frusemide) intravenously.
- Consider giving corticosteroids (see below).
- Give antibiotics after taking blood for bacterial culture and obtaining sputum if possible.

 The basic principles of emergency medical management:
- Stabilize the patient and administer essential initial medication without delay.
- Acquire the knack of doing more than one thing at the same time, e.g. extract details of history while inserting a venous cannula; identify the JVP while a nebulizer is being prepared.

History of the presenting problem

Over what period of time has the exacerbation developed and are there any clues as to its cause? Common contributing factors are:
- Infection—is there anything to suggest an infective process, e.g. fever, purulent sputum or 'flu-like symptoms at the outset?
- Fluid overload—does he have peripheral oedema; could he have suffered an acute myocardial infarction and now be in LVF?
- PE—this is a more common event in chronic airways obstruction than is commonly recognized. Be aware of the possibility. Ask specifically for a history of sudden onset of chest pain, but remember that spontaneous or cough-induced rib fractures occur in chronic airways obstruction, the pain from which can be excruciating and indistinguishable from pleurisy.

Relevant past history

What was the degree of incapacity before the recent deterioration? Make strenuous attempts to determine:
- usual exercise tolerance
- ability to cope with everyday tasks
- general quality of life.

It will be necessary to examine the clinic notes and to speak to relatives as well as interviewing the patient. This information is crucial if respiratory failure becomes inexorable and the appropriateness of assisted ventilation has to be decided.

Examination

How ill is the patient? If he is nearly dead call for help from the ICU immediately.

Does the patient have a pneumothorax? If he does not, proceed to check vital signs—temperature (is he pyrexial?), pulse, blood pressure—and then examine.

Respiratory

What is the pattern of breathing?—is his respiratory rate high, normal or low? Does tidal volume appear relatively normal or is it reduced?

Is there evidence of consolidation? Are there multiple localized crackles? Either suggest infection.

Cardiovascular

Is there any suggestion of fluid overload? The JVP may be elevated because of pulmonary hypertension and, if so, a relatively high venous pressure may be important physiologically in assisting right ventricular function. Nevertheless, pulmonary oedema commonly contributes to an exacerbation of chronic airflow obstruction and it is better to err on the side of giving diuretics rather than failing to treat an element of heart failure.

Are there any symptoms or signs to suggest pulmonary embolism? Listen carefully for a pleural rub. Note that signs of pulmonary hypertension are not useful in arriving at the diagnosis of PE in this context.

Pneumothorax in chronic chest disease

- Even a small air leak on the radiograph can cause severe dyspnoea and distress in a person who has underlying chest disease. An intercostal drain will be indicated most of the time.
- Tension pneumothorax demands immediate drainage—insert a grey venflon through the second intercostal space anteriorly, withdraw the needle and allow air to escape through the cannula—but you must be certain of the diagnosis and in the majority of cases of pneumothorax there will be time to obtain radiograph confirmation.

Approach to investigations and management

Investigations

The following should be requested immediately.

Arterial blood gas analysis

This will tell you how hypoxic the patient is and how effectively he is ventilating; a high $PaCO_2$ indicates diminished alveolar ventilation which may be acute or chronic or a combination of the two (see *Respiratory medicine*, Section 3.6.1).

Chest radiograph

Look specifically for the following:
- pneumothorax
- focal lung pathology—which may be infective consolidation or a bronchial carcinoma
- pulmonary oedema—but note that this can be difficult to diagnose with certainty in the patient with chronic lung disease.

Other blood tests

A full blood count and biochemistry, including blood sugar and cardiac enzymes, is needed. It is vital to know that serum potassium is normal—hypokalaemic respiratory myopathy is a real entity and will compound alveolar hypoventilation.

Electrocardiogram

Determine heart rate and rhythm and look for evidence of ischaemia or of acute myocardial infarction.

Other tests

In individual instances additional investigations will be necessary, e.g. echocardiography, isotope lung scanning (difficult to interpret in chronic lung disease) or CT angiography of the chest.

Management

In a severe exacerbation of chronic airways disease, the following principles apply:
- Antibiotics (see Section 1.9, p. 32 and *Infectious diseases*, Section 1.4) and bronchodilators (see Section 1.7, p. 25) should be given without delay.
- Diuretics will be necessary if there is any evidence of fluid overload.
- Steroids are indicated if wheeze is prominent and many patients with chronic airways disease derive benefit from corticosteroids in an acute exacerbation even if there is no evidence of steroid reversibility when their disease is stable. Generally speaking, it is better to err on the side of giving a stat dose of oral or intravenous steroid in the emergency setting.
- Controlled O_2 (starting with 24%) is administered according to the arterial blood gas findings. Blood gases

should be rechecked regularly to review the effect of your chosen inspired O_2 concentration on hypoxia and to detect progressive hypercapnia in the patient who is a chronic hypoventilator.
• The respiratory stimulant doxapram improves hypercapnic hypoxia (type 2 respiratory failure) in some patients.
• Nasal intermittent positive pressure ventilation (NIPPV) and continuous positive airway pressure (CPAP) are other techniques that can support type 2 respiratory failure [1] (see *Respiratory medicine*, Section 2.12.3).
• Endotracheal intubation and ventilation will be indicated in some patients. This is a complex clinical and ethical issue which is discussed further in the next section.

Formal intubation and ventilation in chronic airways obstruction

Clinical and ethical considerations

Patients with established airways obstruction have a chest wall and diaphragm (the 'respiratory pump') that have been overworked chronically. They fall into two types:
• the 'pink puffer'—where the respiratory pump continues to work overtime in an effort to maintain normoxia
• the 'blue bloater'—who has relative pump failure and hypoventilates, with hypercapnic hypoxia as the result.

If an acute respiratory exacerbation refractory to the treatment measures described above occurs in either case and the patient is then placed on mechanical ventilation, the respiratory pump is given a holiday, which it considers well deserved. Adequate gas exchange is ensured by the mechanical ventilator, but problems start when attempts are made to wean the patient from assisted ventilation—the chronically tired respiratory pump is reluctant to take up the demand (Fig. 23).

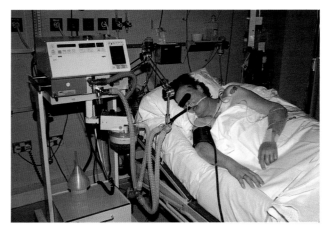

Fig. 23 Problems start when the time comes to wean the patient from assisted ventilation.

Before crossing the rubicon to assisted ventilation in patients with chronic airways disease, there should be a calculated and comprehensive assessment of their ability to restore effective, physiological ventilation when the cause of the acute exacerbation has been treated. This calculation requires consideration of several salient factors:
• What was the patient's exercise tolerance and general quality of life before the acute illness?
• Is there evidence from hospital records of the severity of the chest disease prior to the acute deterioration? (Fig. 24).
• Is there evidence of significant reversibility of the airways obstruction? Information from previous reversibility tests with bronchodilators and steroids will be important.
• Has assisted ventilation been successful in the past?
• Has the deterioration been precipitated by an obvious acute event, which could be pneumonia, severe fluid overload or PE?

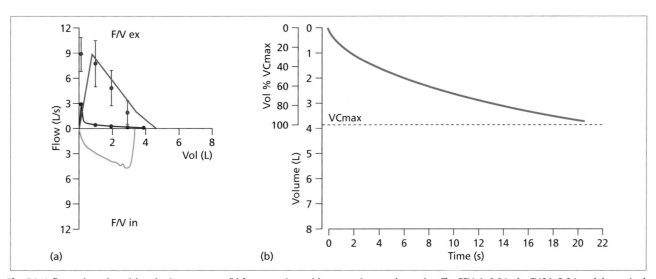

Fig. 24 A flow-volume loop (a) and spirogram trace (b) from a patient with severe airways obstruction. The FEV_1 is 0.8 L, the FVC is 3.8 L and the expired limb of the flow-volume loop shows the classical 'elbow' of collapsible airways obstruction. The diagnosis of emphysema is virtually confirmed.

- Alternatively, does the evidence point to a gradual, inexorable decline in respiratory function?

Medical records are of paramount importance; so is information from medical and nursing staff who have cared for the patient in the past. Consultant opinion must be sought if at all possible before deciding that endotracheal intubation and ventilation are the correct steps for an individual patient.

See *General clinical issues*, Section 3; *Respiratory medicine*, Sections 1.15 and 2.11.
Shneerson J. *Handbook of Sleep Medicine*. Oxford: Blackwell Science, 2000.

1.11 Upper gastrointestinal haemorrhage

Case history

The ambulance service contacts the Emergency Medical department in your hospital to inform them that a man in his sixties is being rushed in by 'blue-light' ambulance after suffering a major gastrointestinal haemorrhage. The ambulance crew are concerned because he is hypotensive, cold and clammy. They found him in a pool of fresh blood that he had vomited when they arrived at his home following a 999 call. Nursing staff in the emergency department call you to be ready to receive this patient as you are the physician on medical intake for the day.

Clinical approach

The nursing staff have been prudent in calling you early. When a patient requires resuscitation and you have foreknowledge of this, plan your strategy:
- Organize staff and decide on individual duties.
- Prepare intravenous lines, drug infusions and equipment.
- Request a search for hospital records.

This is a basic plan: but how often do delays occur for lack of preparation in the emergency situation?

The patient arrives, you have no previous history, the patient is unaccompanied and the Records Department has been unable to find previous hospital notes.

The immediate priorities are haemodynamic assessment, venous access and giving fluid.

Haemodynamic assessment

Note the following:
- Is the patient shut down peripherally? Check fingers,

toes and nose. How far up the arm or leg do you have to go until they feel warm?
- Identifying and measuring the JVP is often difficult but it is one of the most vital of physical signs. A low JVP is the most reliable indicator of volume depletion.
- Blood pressure can be measured electronically but should be checked manually: remember that it is important to measure postural fall in pressure, detailing measurements, '110/60 lying; 80/50 sitting', as well as measuring paradox in the patient who has collapsed.
- A compensatory rise in pulse rate may not accompany volume depletion in the elderly or if there is autonomic neuropathy for any reason, e.g. diabetes.

 Assessing haemodynamic status

The JVP:
- Make a point of looking for the venous pressure in all your patients; familiarity with the normal wave-form helps enormously in recognizing the abnormal.
- It is not good enough to comment 'JVP not elevated'; it must be measured from the angle of Louis and if not seen at 45 degrees then the patient should be tilted up or down until it can be detected, ' +10 cm at 90 degrees' … 'visible only when lying flat' and so on.

Postural hypotension:
- Postural hypotension is often the straw that breaks the camel's back: how many times have you heard—'he said he was alright, but when he got up he nearly fainted and I had to call the doctor'?
- A blood pressure when lying down of 110/60 might be normal, but if it falls when the patient sits up, then it is not.

Venous access

Practical considerations:
- Insert large cannulae into both antecubital fossae.
- If access is difficult, insert a femoral venous line by Seldinger technique. If you cannot do this—get someone who can.
- Do not attempt immediate cannulation into a neck vein in a collapsed, hypovolaemic patient—the veins are constricted in volume depletion, rendering the procedure difficult and much more liable to complication as you use the 'sewing machine technique' (multiple stabs) in increasing desperation. A central line never made anyone better, but has killed in this situation.

 Do not believe the doctor who claims never to have failed when performing a particular practical procedure. He just hasn't done enough!

Intravenous fluids

Give fluid that remains in the intravascular compartment:
- Colloid.
- Saline.

• O negative blood, if in extremis. This is rarely necessary, as an emergency cross match (infinitely safer) should be achievable in 20–30 min.
• Do not give dextrose or dextrose–saline: the dextrose is rapidly metabolized leaving free water which seeps out of the vascular space.

The rate of delivery is important:
• Give 1 L of fluid as fast as possible.
• Repeat examination of JVP and blood pressure.

If JVP is low and postural hypotension persists:
• Give 1 L of fluid as fast as possible.
• Repeat until the JVP is raised to the upper limit of normal and postural hypotension is abolished.

Monitoring fluid balance

Insert a catheter to monitor urinary output: if this is poor do not continue to infuse fluid when the venous pressure has risen or you will induce fluid overload and pulmonary oedema.

History of the presenting problem

With emergency measures completed, continue clinical assessment of the patient. Important features of the history are discussed below.

Are there clues as to the cause and source of the bleeding?

A history of previous peptic ulceration is important and so is an existing prescription for NSAIDs.

Enquire regarding alcohol intake and other risk factors for cirrhosis (see *General clinical issues*, Section 2). Remember that upper GI bleeding in the setting of alcohol abuse is often caused by pathology other than oesophageal or gastric varices.

Examination

Clinical examination, after assessment of the circulation as detailed above, should not be restricted to the abdominal findings.

General

Are there signs suggestive of iron deficiency anaemia: smooth tongue, angular stomatitis and koilonychia (the latter is easier felt than seen when in its early stages)?

Are there signs of chronic liver disease or of portal hypertension? (Fig. 25 and Table 7).

Is Virchow's node enlarged and craggy? If so the diagnosis of gastrointestinal malignancy is virtually secure.

Table 7 Signs of liver disease.

Signs of chronic liver disease	Signs of portal hypertension	Signs of hepatic encephalopathy
Spider naevi	Splenomegaly	Myoclonus: the 'liver flap'
Palmar erythema	Caput medusae	Hepatic foetor
Leuconychia	Ascites	
Bruising		
Gynaecomastia		
Testicular atrophy		
Clubbing (rarely)		

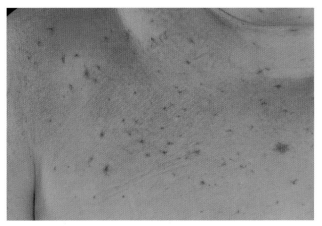

Fig. 25 Spider naevi in a patient with alcohol-induced cirrhosis.

Abdominal

Some clinical signs suggest that bleeding is continuing:
• A stomach full of blood is uncomfortable and the patient will find epigastric palpation unpleasant.
• Blood stimulates intestinal motility and bowel sounds are usually very active on auscultation.

The absence of these two observations is reassuring that active bleeding has ceased, but they are not infallible.

The presence of an abdominal mass may indicate gastric malignancy, and peritonism may point to a peptic ulcer that has perforated as well as bled (although this is rare).

Always perform a rectal examination: the colour and smell of melaena are unmistakeable.

Approach to investigations and management

Investigations

The following should be requested as emergency investigations.

Blood tests

Arrange emergency cross match (4 units are usually enough to start with). Check full blood count, electrolytes, renal and liver function tests and clotting.

Table 8 Risk scoring system for acute upper gastrointestinal (GI) bleeding [2].

Score	0	1	2	3
Age	<60 years	60–79 years	>80 years	
Shock	No shock	Pulse >100 Systolic BP >100	Systolic BP<100	
Comorbidity	None		Cardiac failure, ischaemic heart disease, other major comorbidity	Renal failure, liver failure, widespread malignancy
Diagnosis	Mallory–Weiss or no lesion seen	All other diagnoses	Malignancy of upper GI tract	
Major stigmata of recent haemorrhage at endoscopy	None or dark spot only		Blood in upper GI tract, adherent clot visible or spurting vessel	

Remember that a relatively normal haemoglobin does not exclude significant haemorrhage; there may have been insufficient time for haemodilution to have taken place. An iron deficient picture suggests acute or chronic blood loss.

Radiological tests

The chest can be radiographed portably and, if the film is taken with the patient upright, it can help to exclude perforation of a viscus as well as aspiration.

An abdominal film, by contrast, will require a trip to the radiograph department and this may not be advisable for an unstable patient. An abdominal film is extremely unlikely to provide additional diagnostic help in gastrointestinal bleeding if there is no evidence of concomitant peritonism or intestinal obstruction: do not ask for one unless these are plausible diagnoses.

Management

Gastrointestinal bleeding—a team game:
• If haemorrhage is profuse, continuing or recurrent then early surgical opinion is manadatory.

Risk scoring in upper gastrointestinal haemorrhage

Consider the following points, each of which has a bearing on prognosis and mortality risk:
• Haematemesis is a more serious symptom than melaena. Mortality rises from 5% in patients suffering melaena with clear nasogastric aspirate to 12% in those with melaena and fresh blood in the nasogastric aspirate.
• Patients passing red blood per rectum with fresh blood in the nasogastric aspirate are reported to have a mortality rate of 29% [1].
• Older patients with GI haemorrhage have a higher mortality and you must be alert to the need for surgical treatment, particularly in the elderly who continue to bleed or who rebleed.

A combination of clinical features and endoscopic findings has provided a numerical scoring system of risk in upper GI haemorrhage (Table 8). The maximum additive score prior to diagnosis by endoscopy is 7. Mortality is as follows:
• score 0 = 0.2%
• score 1 = 2.4%
• score 2 = 5.6%
• score 3 = 11%
• score 4 = 25%
• score 5 = 40%
• score 6 or 7 = 50%.
Mortality of all patients who rebleed in hospital is 40%.

Varices

Bleeding oesophageal varices can cause torrential loss of blood. Get help from the specialist gastroenterological/ hepatological team immediately if this is likely to be the diagnosis, i.e. bleeding in a patient known to have varices, or bleeding in a patient who seems particularly likely to have varices.

Urgent endoscopy (Fig. 26) is mandatory—banding or sclerotherapy can be attempted during the procedure.

Consider giving terlipressin (2 mg i.v., followed by 1 or 2 mg every 4–6 h until bleeding is controlled, for up to 72 h) which can reduce portal blood pressure.

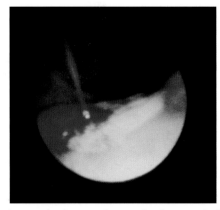

Fig. 26 A photograph taken at endoscopy showing a peptic ulcer with a spurting artery. An obvious case for intervention!

Have a Sengstaken tube available—but this should only be introduced by those with experience of the technique.

Gastrointestinal bleeding

- Resuscitate.
- Can you determine the cause of the bleeding?
- Is there evidence that bleeding is continuing? Urgent upper gastrointestinal endoscopy is mandatory and offers therapeutic options as well as being the diagnostic investigation of choice.
- Do you require a surgical opinion? Massive haemorrhage or the patient who rebleeds in hospital are two groups that certainly need this.

See *Gastroenterology*, Sections 1.3, 2.3 and 2.10.
1 Silverstein FE, Gilbert DA, Tedesco FJ *et al.* The national ASGE survey on upper gastrointestinal bleeding: II. Clinical prognostic factors. *Gastrointest Endosc* 1981; 27: 80–93.
2 Rockall TA, Logan RFA, Devlin HB *et al.* Risk assessment after acute upper gastrointestinal haemorrhage. *Gut* 1996; 38: 316–321.

1.12 Bloody diarrhoea

Case history

A woman of 37 years has suffered 48 h of frequent watery diarrhoea; blood has been mixed with the motions for the past 24 h during which time she has had her bowels open 10 times. She has been diagnosed as having inflammatory bowel disease but her bowel symptoms are normally well controlled with a regular prescription for Salazopyrin and rectal administration of steroids. Her general practitioner's letter mentions that the patient and her husband had entertained friends at an evening barbecue 3 days before the diarrhoea started.

Clinical approach

The two commonest causes of bloody diarrhoea are colonic infection and inflammatory bowel disease. The immediate priorities are discussed below.

Check vital signs

- Check airway, breathing and carefully assess the cardiovascular findings.
- Hypovolaemia and the circulatory consequences of sepsis are potential sequelae of a presentation such as this.

- Pulse, blood pressure, JVP, signs of peripheral perfusion and core temperature (with a tympanic thermometer in this case) should be recorded.

Abdominal

Find out:
- Is there evidence of peritonism?
- Is the abdomen distended?
- Can an abdominal mass be felt?
- The presence or absence of bowel sounds should be noted. Do they sound obstructive?

Ask for an urgent surgical opinion if any of these features are present.

A rectal examination is mandatory:
- Inspect the perineum first, looking for skin changes or fistulae suggestive of Crohn's disease.
- Search the rectum for a possible mass.
- Examine any faeces on your gloved finger for melaena or frank blood.

Resuscitate

Obtain intravenous access and administer appropriate intravenous fluids as quickly as is necessary to correct hypovolaemia (see Section 1.11, p. 39).

Urgent investigations

Blood tests

These should include full blood count, renal and liver function tests, serum albumin, C-reactive protein, erythrocyte sedimentation rate (ESR) and blood cultures (see below under Approach to investigations and management).

Radiology

An erect chest radiograph should include the hemidiaphragms to look for evidence of perforation (Fig. 27). A supine abdominal film should be taken to exclude toxic dilatation and look for other prognostic radiological signs of inflammatory bowel disease (Fig. 28 and Table 9).

Stool

Faeces should be sent for microbiological investigation (microscopy, culture and specific testing for *Clostridium difficile* toxin). The sample can be obtained during sigmoidoscopy if the patient has not opened their bowels before this is performed.

Nocturnal diarrhoea is sometimes quoted as a poor prognostic feature but, in fact, this feature is most useful as an indicator of organic pathology and in distinguishing

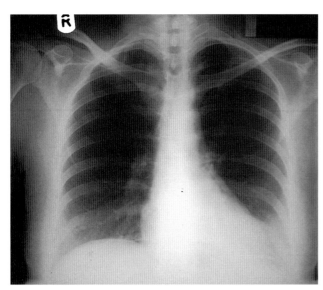

Fig. 27 Chest radiograph showing air under both hemidiaphragms. No apologies for the subtle changes—they are often as subtle in real life!

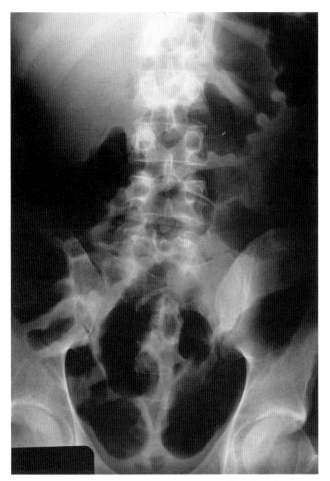

Fig. 28 Abdominal radiograph in acute ulcerative colitis. The colon is dilated (not quite to 10 cm but worrying nonetheless). Thumb-printing of colonic mucosa is seen in the left upper abdomen and there are dilated loops of small bowel.

Table 9 Findings that ring alarm bells in acute ulcerative colitis.

Bowels open 9–12 times in the first 24 h
Pulse >100 beats/min
Fever >38°C
Albumin <30 g/L
CRP >45 mg/L
Mucosal islands, toxic megacolon and dilated small bowel on abdominal radiograph

CRP, C-reactive protein.

from the irritable bowel syndrome rather than pointing to severity in acute inflammatory bowel disease.

Sigmoidoscopy

Sigmoidoscopy provides useful diagnostic information (Fig. 29). It should be performed after the abdominal radiograph because enthusiastic introduction of air during the procedure can produce a picture alarmingly similar to toxic dilatation!
• Normal rectal mucosa usually excludes active ulcerative colitis (although this woman has been taking a rectal steroid preparation, which can diminish the superficial appearances of inflammation).
• Inflamed rectal mucosa can be a feature of any cause of severe diarrhoea.
• The presence of contact bleeding, ulceration or the pseudomembrane of antibiotic-associated pseudomembranous colitis are more specific.
• A rectal biopsy should be taken below the peritoneal reflection, i.e. within 10 cm of the anal margin.

 Acute colitis
• Assessment of the cardiovascular system is as important as the abdominal findings.
• Correct hypovolaemia and beware the toxic patient.
• Exclude peritonism and any clinical evidence (abdominal or systemic) of toxic dilatation of the colon. If either are present arrange surgical review immediately.
• Early sigmoidoscopy (with a rectal biopsy) is important.
• Organize laboratory tests and radiographs to exclude bad prognostic features and complications of acute inflammatory bowel disease.

History of the presenting problem

After the immediate priorities have been addressed, or in those who are less severely ill, proceed to obtain details of the following.

Intensity and nature of the diarrhoea

 Diarrhoea is difficult to define but easy to recognize if you have it!

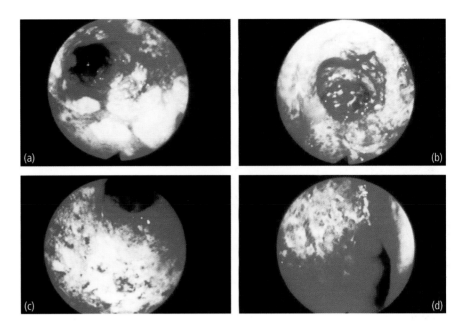

Fig. 29 Sigmoidoscopic appearances of ulcerative colitis, showing inflamed mucosa, ulceration and contact bleeding.

Has the patient got diarrhoea at all? A careful history is necessary if you are to be certain that diarrhoea is genuinely present. Most authorities agree with the definition of 'more than 200 g of stool in 24 h', but different patients use the term to describe different things. How many times have they opened their bowels today? If they have been in the medical admissions unit for several hours without needing a bedpan, then they are unlikely to be 'going every hour'.

The nature of the diarrhoea is important in diagnosis. Frequent passage of small amounts of stool implies different pathology from the situation where very large volumes are being passed. Proctitis or a rectal lesion is likely in the former situation and small-bowel pathology in the latter.

A history of bloody diarrhoea is highly suggestive of colonic pathology, whereas copious bulky stools, foul-smelling and difficult to flush away are characteristic of malabsorption.

Were there any obvious precipitating factors?

Contaminated or infected food is an obvious culprit in this case, but also ask about medication.
• Has there been a recent prescription of antibiotics? These predispose to *Clostridium difficile*.
• Are NSAIDs taken regularly? These are a potent cause of colonic irritation and bloody diarrhoea.

Clues to specific intestinal infections in the patient presenting with diarrhoea are shown in Table 10.

Previous history of bowel problems

Is there a record of:
• A diagnosis of inflammatory bowel disease, as in this case? (Remember that a colonic neoplasm is a possibility in long-standing ulcerative colitis.)
• Bowel surgery?
• Abdominal irradiation?—'radiation colitis' can present with bloody diarrhoea.

Is there other relevant pathology?

The sudden onset of pain and bloody diarrhoea in an elderly arteriopath should alert you to the possibility of ischaemic colitis. Do they have a history or findings to suggest atherosclerotic vascular disease?

Social and sexual history

Has the patient been abroad? If they have, a wider differential of intestinal infections (Table 10) needs to be considered.

HIV-related bowel infections, particularly cytomegalovirus, may present in this way. In appropriate circumstances you will need to enquire about this (see *General clinical issues*, Section 2).

Examination

The important points are:
• Assess fluid balance.
• Look for fever and other evidence of sepsis.
• Is the patient anaemic?
• Is there peripheral oedema?—likely, with a low venous pressure, to indicate hypoproteinaemia due to acute/chronic bowel inflammation in this case.
• What are the findings on abdominal examination?
• Examine the perineum and rectum and perform a sigmoidoscopy with rectal biopsy.

Site of infection	Infectious agent	Predisposing cause
Small bowel infection	Cholera	? Foreign travel
	Enterotoxigenic *E. coli*	Infected meat
	Rotavirus Norwalk virus Small round virus	Common and associated with vomiting
	Toxin production *Staph. aureus*	Symptoms a few hours after ingestion of contaminated material. Vomiting associated
	Toxin production *Bacillus cereus*	Classically associated with contaminated rice and accompanied by vomiting
Colonic infection	*Campylobacter jejuni*	Commonest in the UK today. Beware of undercooked chicken.
	Shigella and *Salmonella*	Classical cause of dysentery and associated with bloody diarrhoea
	Amoebiasis	Can be contracted in UK, so an important consideration on acute medical 'intake'
	Clostridium difficile	Associated with antibiotic therapy. Toxin-producing
	Enterohaemorrhagic *E. coli*	Produces a shiga-like toxin and potential complications are haemolytic–uraemic syndrome and thrombotic thrombocytopaenic purpura

Table 10 Intestinal infections.

Physiology of the bowel

The daily dietary intake of food and liquid, combined with gastric and intestinal secretions, results in a volume load of approximately 7 L for the small intestine.

By the time intestinal contents have reached the terminal ileum only about 1.5 L remains: hence, when there is small-bowel pathology there is often large-volume diarrhoea.

Approach to investigations and management

Investigations

The strategy for urgent investigation has been described above but note the following:
• Anaemia may be acute if bleeding is profuse and there has been time for haemodilution, but it is more likely to indicate chronic pathology, e.g. poorly controlled inflammatory bowel disease or a coexisting haematological condition.
• The blood film and haematological indices are important: microcytic, hypochromic changes are likely to indicate blood loss, whereas macrocytosis points to malabsorption or alcohol abuse.
• A slight elevation in white cell count is of little help in differential diagnosis but, if elevated beyond 15 000, be alerted to the possibility of sepsis.

• A serum albumin of less than 30 g/L is a bad feature in inflammatory bowel disease because albumin loss is proportional to the extent of bowel involvement. It is particularly worrying in acute ulcerative colitis.
• The C-reactive protein is useful clinically. If it is elevated (>45 mg/L) in ulcerative colitis, the patient is sick. On the other hand, its elevation in an acute exacerbation of Crohn's disease (the disease produces more of an acute phase response) is not quite so worrying.
• Consider and investigate unusual infections, e.g. *Yersinia* colitis with *Yersinia* antibodies.

Overwhelming sepsis can be present in a patient who is apyrexial and with a normal white cell count.

Be aware of the poor prognostic features of acute ulcerative colitis (see Table 9).

Management

The immediate priorities have been described above:
• Resuscitate—correct volume depletion vigorously.
• Be alert to the toxic patient—if there are signs of sepsis, serious haemodynamic disturbance and/or abnormal

abdominal findings that suggest perforation or toxic mega-colon, seek urgent surgical advice.

Other issues

Antibiotics

In all cases of acute colitis be aware of the possibility of bowel infection: the chronic colitic is perfectly entitled to contract *Campylobacter* (as in this case study). Blood and stool cultures should always be taken—but in the patient who is very ill, if you cannot exclude infection, then it is safer to treat empirically with a combination of ciprofloxacin and metronidazole. This will cover most potential pathogens, including amoebae and *Clostridium difficile*.

Could the patient have pseudomembranous colitis? Many antibiotics are associated with this condition, particularly third-generation cephalosporins. Treat with metronidazole or vancomycin after sigmoidoscopy (and rectal biopsy) has been performed and stool has been sent for *Clostridium difficile* toxin.

Steroids

A moderate or severe exacerbation of inflammatory bowel disease should be treated with systemic steroids (methylprednisolone 80–120 mg i.v. per day given in two divided doses). Less severe exacerbations (perhaps limited to the rectum) may be appropriately managed with rectal steroid preparations, with or without a smaller dose of oral or intravenous steroid. 5-ASA products may have a role in the acute attack.

Important to note

The patient described in the case history suffered an episode of *Campylobacter* infection and responded to ciprofloxacin. The possibility of an exacerbation of inflammatory bowel disease was covered initially with corticosteroids until positive stool cultures secured the diagnosis.

 See *Gastroenterology*, Sections 1.1, 1.5, 1.11 and 2.1.
DuPont HL. Guidelines on acute infectious diarrhoea in adults. *Am J Gastroenterol* 1997; 92: 1962–1975.
Greenstein AJ, Aufses AH. Differences in pathogenesis, incidence and outcome of perforation in inflammatory bowel disease. *Surg Gynaecol Obstet* 1985; 160: 63–69.
Iveson TJ, Chan A. Pseudomembranous colitis complicating chemotherapy. *Lancet* 1992; 339: 192–193.
Sheth SG, LaMont JT. Toxic megacolon. *Lancet* 1998; 351: 509–513.

1.13 'The medical abdomen'

Patients with acute abdominal pain are usually admitted under the surgical team ... but, for a variety of reasons, not always! The physician needs to be wary of the surgical acute abdomen that has been incorrectly referred and also aware of conditions such as pancreatitis and biliary tract disease where joint medical and surgical management can be beneficial.

Case history

A young woman in her twenties is admitted with severe right upper quadrant pain and a fever.

Clinical approach

The important issues are discussed below.

General

• Is the cardiovascular system compromised? If so, resuscitate immediately (see Section 1.11, p. 38).
• Is there evidence of sepsis, either generalized or localized to the abdomen?

Abdominal

• Is there evidence of peritonism or of intestinal obstruction?
• Are there localized abdominal findings, e.g. local tenderness with or without a mass, an enlarged organ, perhaps a pyonephrosis or an empyema of the gall bladder in this case?
• Are the bowel sounds normal or do they sound obstructed? Is there complete silence, suggesting peritonitis?
• Always examine the hernial orifices—remember to look in 'unusual sites', e.g. periumbilical. A strangulated hernia may be accompanied by trophic change in the overlying skin.
• Rectal examination may reveal hard stool in the elderly, compacted and obstructed patient; or the rectum may be empty as in small bowel obstruction. Tenderness in the right iliac fossa on rectal examination is common in appendicitis.

History of the presenting problem

There are three main causes of abdominal pain: visceral, parietal and referred. Which is most prominent? And what is the likely explanation? The key questions are discussed below.

What does the pain feel like?

Constant, generalized and severe

Constant, generalized, severe pain, exacerbated by any movement, is highly suggestive of peritonitis.

Colicky

Colicky pain is likely to be visceral in origin and its characteristics should help to decide which organ is responsible: regular waves of colicky pain, which become increasingly severe and then diminish, which are fairly generalized but may be periumbilical in site are the hallmarks of small intestinal obstruction. Longer lived episodes of pain with less of a crescendo–decrescendo pattern and maximal in the right upper quadrant will point to biliary tract disease. The pain of renal colic is often more prolonged, sited in one or other flank and with typical radiation around to the anterior abdomen and down into the inguinal region, perhaps terminating in the scrotum in men or in the area of the labium majoris in women.

Where is the pain and does it radiate?

The site where visceral pain is experienced depends upon the intestinal segment involved:
• Oesophageal pain is often in the epigastrium or low central chest.
• Duodenal pain is felt in the epigastrium or just to the right of it.
• Small bowel pain is poorly localized and is generally felt diffusely in the periumbilical region.
• Colonic pain usually occurs in roughly the area in which the diseased colonic segment lies; this is also true of terminal ileal pathology.
• Gall-bladder pain is most commonly felt in the right upper quadrant but rarely it can be exclusively left sided and this odd presentation is quite unexplained.
• Pancreatic pain is sited in the epigastrium but there is often a lot of associated discomfort in the lumbar region of the back. In addition, pancreatitis is a potential cause of generalized abdominal pain and can mimic the peritonism of a ruptured viscus.

How long has the pain been present and how did it start?

Most causes of abdominal pain start gradually, but perforation of a viscus can occasionally cause sudden pain.

Are there relieving or exacerbating features?

Parietal pain is exacerbated by even slight movement, which explains why patients with peritonitis lie perfectly still. By contrast, the patient with visceral pain often writhes around in an attempt to find a more comfortable position when a spasm of pain attacks.
• Pain which is aggravated by tension or anxiety is a feature of irritable bowel syndrome.
• Relief of pain by food is a strong pointer to peptic ulceration.
• Exacerbation by food, on the other hand, implies an obstructive component, gastritis or oesophagitis.
• Gastric or duodenal inflammation is associated with alcohol, aspirin and other NSAIDs.
• Diffuse abdominal pain appearing 20 min to 1 hour after meals raises the possibility of intestinal angina.
• The pain of duodenal ulceration is typically severe in the early hours of the morning and there may be a definite periodicity to the pain, e.g. nightly bouts of pain for a few weeks followed by a symptom-free period.
• Oesophageal pain is typically exacerbated by posture, bending or stooping.

How long does the pain last?

Severe acute pain persisting for several hours often implies catastrophic events such as perforation, strangulation or intestinal obstruction. Biliary pain becomes progressively more intense with time but can be relieved suddenly with the passage of a stone, leaving a dull, aching sensation in the right upper quadrant.

Is the pain referred?

Pain may be referred from visceral organs or parietal peritoneum to areas innervated from the same dermatome:
• Oesophageal pain may radiate to the neck or arms.
• Pain from the distal colon may refer to the lumbar spine.
• Gall-bladder pain radiates classically to the right infrascapular region. An area of hyperaesthesia can exist over the referred area and this can be helpful in gall-bladder disease when heightened sensation over the lower border of the scapula supports the diagnosis.
• Pain from a duodenal ulcer which radiates through to the back usually indicates penetration of the ulcer into the pancreas.

Be wary of thoracic pathology masquerading as an acute abdomen. Pleurisy from either side, particularly when the lower pleural surfaces are involved, can result in referred pain in one or other upper quadrant. Add to this the fact that 'sympathetic' pleural effusions and even lower zone pulmonary consolidation can accompany abdominal pathology in the upper quadrant (the classic example is a subphrenic abscess) and the potential for diagnostic confusion becomes clear!

Approach to investigations and management

Investigations

The emergency investigations discussed below need to be ordered.

Blood tests

FULL BLOOD COUNT

Anaemia may be due to acute blood loss or it may be a result of underlying (and perhaps associated) disease. Pay attention to MCV and MCHC and to the blood film. Neutrophilia supports the presence of sepsis.

ELECTROLYTES, RENAL AND LIVER FUNCTION TESTS

Look for hypokalaemia and renal failure. Liver function tests may help diagnostically.

SERUM AMYLASE

Serum amylase should be checked without fail.

Radiological tests

SUPINE ABDOMINAL RADIOGRAPH

A supine abdominal radiograph may diagnose intestinal obstruction (and perhaps perforation) or help to localize pathology, e.g. the dilated contiguous loop of bowel in cholecystitis; the pattern of bowel dilatation seen with sigmoid volvulus; the classical appearances of toxic megacolon.

CHEST RADIOGRAPH

An erect or semi-erect chest radiograph is more efficient at diagnosing perforation and has the advantage of being possible with a portable radiograph machine (see Section 1.12, Fig. 27, p. 42).

ABDOMINAL CT SCAN

An abdominal CT scan should not delay laparotomy in the patient with obvious peritonitis, but is a very useful and increasingly used investigation (Fig. 30).

Management

The approach to management can be summarized as follows:
• Correct intravascular volume depletion vigorously with saline, colloid or blood as appropriate (see Section 1.11, p. 39).

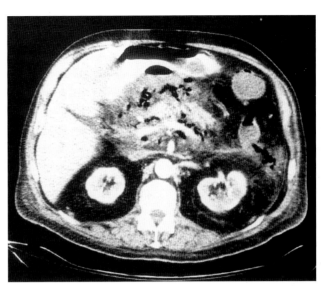

Fig. 30 CT scan showing necrotizing pancreatitis with gas formation. The pain was identical to that of peritonitis.

• Broad-spectrum antibiotics must be given promptly if there is any evidence of sepsis.
• Seek surgical help early when appropriate.
• Remember 'medical' causes of the acute abdomen, e.g. shingles (without the rash yet!), porphyria, diabetic ketoacidosis, sickle-cell crisis and familial Mediterranean fever—but if in doubt, bet on a common condition.

 Common things are commonest.

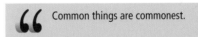 See *Gastroenterology*, Section 1.9.
Glasgow RE, Mulvihill SJ. Abdominal pain, including the acute abdomen. In: Feldman M, Sleisenger MH, Scharschmidt BF, eds. *Gastrointestinal and Liver Disease. Pathophysiology, Diagnosis, Management* (6th edn). Philadelphia: Saunders, 1998, vol. 1, pp. 80–89.

1.14 Hepatic encephalopathy/ alcohol withdrawal

Case history

A 55-year-old man is brought to A&E having been found confused and shaking in the street. He is a regular attender in the department and is a known alcoholic.

Clinical approach

Your main concern in any alcoholic patient who presents with confusion and tremor is to exclude any serious or life-threatening condition. Do not assume that the patient is just drunk—this is a dangerous thing to do,

Table 11 Differential diagnosis of confusion in a known alcoholic.

Alcohol intoxication
Acute alcohol withdrawal
Delirium tremens
Hepatic encephalopathy
Hypoglycaemia
Head injury
Subdural haematoma
Wernicke's encephalopathy
Any severe illness, particularly sepsis

both for you and for the patient. Acute liver failure is a medical emergency and requires immediate treatment. Consider the differential diagnosis shown in Table 11.

History of the presenting problem

Although the patient may not be able to give a coherent history, information gained from friends or relatives and previous hospital notes may help to determine the cause of the acute problem.

Ask the following:
• How much alcohol does he usually drink? Has he stopped over the past few days or has he been on a 'bender'?
• Has there been a recent head injury?
• Is there a history of liver disease? If so, ask about possible causes of acute decompensation, e.g. recent infections, haematemesis, alcohol binges or constipation.
• Drug history. Ask specifically about drugs that may cause liver failure, e.g. paracetemol overdose, phenytoin, sulphonamides and drugs which may cause decompensation of chronic liver disease, e.g. benzodiazepines.

Examination

General

• What does the patient look and smell like? If he smells of alcohol then acute withdrawal is unlikely, but you cannot exclude other serious problems.
• Assess his conscious level (GCS) and look for any signs of a tremor or asterixis (liver flap).
• Look for signs of chronic liver disease, e.g. jaundice, bruising, spider naevi, Dupytren's contracture, liver palms and scratch marks (Fig. 31).
• Check his temperature.
• Remember to look carefully at the head for any signs of injury.

Cardiovascular assessment

Check the pulse and blood pressure. Tachycardia and hypertension are seen in acute alcohol withdrawal and delirium tremens. Acute liver failure may cause hypotension.

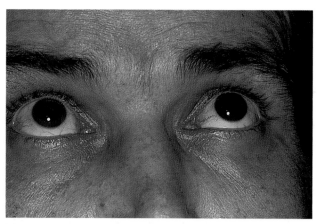

(a)

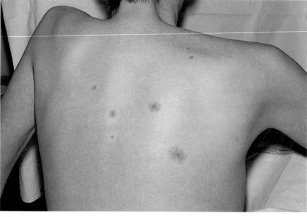

(b)

Fig. 31 Signs of chronic liver disease. (a) Yellow sclera in a patient with jaundice. (b) Spider naevi in a patient with cirrhosis. (From Axford J. *Medicine*. Oxford: Blackwell Science, 1996, with permission.)

Respiratory assessment

Listen specifically for signs of chest infection or pulmonary oedema.

Abdominal assessment

Look for abdominal tenderness, hepatomegaly (unlikely in chronic liver disease), splenomegaly and ascites.

Neurological assessment

Use the GCS, but if hepatic encephalopathy is suspected, what is the grade (Table 12)?

Table 12 Grades of hepatic encephalopathy.

Grade 1	Mildly drowsy but coherent; mood change, impaired concentration and psychomotor function
Grade 2	Drowsy, confused, but able to answer questions
Grade 3	Very drowsy but rousable; alternatively incoherent and agitated
Grade 4a	Responsive only to painful stimuli
Grade 4b	Unresponsive

Check eye movements—looking for opthalmoplegia or gaze palsy. Are there any focal neurological signs?

Approach to investigations and management

Investigations

Pulse oximetry—is the man hypoxic?

Blood tests

• Check U & Es, LFTs, glucose, phosphate, FBC and coagulation screen.
• Do arterial blood gases (arterial ammonia concentration recommended by some).
• Send blood cultures.
• In a case of unexplained acute liver failure (but not this case) check paracetamol level and send blood for viral hepatitis serology and autoantibodies.

Urine tests

Send urine for microscopy, culture and sensitivity.

Chest radiograph

Look for evidence of infection and pulmonary oedema.

Ascitic fluid

Send a sample of ascitic fluid for microscopy and culture: bacterial peritonitis is common in decompensated chronic liver disease.

Immediate investigations of a patient with acute liver failure should include:
• BM stix to exclude hypoglycaemia.
• LFTs and U & Es to confirm diagnosis and detect electrolyte disturbance and renal impairment.
• Prothrombin time to detect potential bleeding problems.
• Blood cultures, urine culture and chest radiograph to look for an infective cause of decompensation.

Management

Acute liver failure and hepatic encephalopathy

SUPPORTIVE MEASURES

These include:
• Give O₂ and monitor O₂ saturation—intubation and ventilation may be required in severe hepatic encephalopathy.

• Ensure adequate intravenous access—if hypovolaemic, give colloid. Note that hyponatraemia (if present) is due to water excess and not to sodium deficiency and should not be treated with infusion of 0.9% (normal) saline.
• Put in a nasogastric tube. Adequate nutrition is important and drugs can be given reliably by this route.
• Give ranitidine 50 mg i.v. slowly to reduce the risk of stress ulceration.

TREATMENT OF METABOLIC ABNORMALITIES

Treat electrolyte and metabolic abnormalities promptly:
• Correct hypokalaemia.
• If hypoglycaemic, give i.v. glucose to maintain BM >3.5 mmol/L.
• If serum phosphate is low start intravenous or oral replacement therapy.

 If there is a history of chronic alcohol intake or malnourishment give thiamine i.v. before glucose to avoid precipitating Wernicke's encephalopathy.

REDUCTION OF INTESTINAL NITROGENOUS LOAD

• Start lactulose 20–30 mL tds or lactitol 10 g tds. Reduce dose when diarrhoea starts.
• Give a phosphate enema.
• Consider giving neomycin or metronidazole if the patient is poorly responsive or comatose.

TREATMENT OF COAGULOPATHY

• Give vitamin K orally or intravenously.
• Consider giving fresh frozen plasma or platelets if actively bleeding, but only after senior haematological advice.

TREATMENT OF UNDERLYING INFECTION

Start broad-spectrum antibiotics (e.g. ceftriaxone or cefotaxime 2 g i.v.) if infection is suspected. Remember that bacterial peritonitis occurs in around 25% of patients with cirrhotic ascites.

VITAMIN SUPPLEMENTATION

Vitamins B and C are usually deficient in chronic alcoholics.
• If consciousness is impaired give Pabrinex i.v. 2–3 pairs 8-hourly. Remember this may cause anaphylaxis.
• If the patient can tolerate oral therapy start oral thiamine (50 mg od), vitamin B tablets compound strong (1–2 tablets tds) and vitamin C (100 mg od).

TREATMENT OF COMPLICATIONS

• Renal failure may complicate liver failure. Consider haemofiltration.
• Cerebral oedema may occur in acute liver failure but is said to be rare in patients with cirrhosis. Consider giving mannitol 200 mg/kg i.v. slowly. Intracranial pressure monitoring can be useful but is not available in all centres.

Note that the development of complications means a very poor prognosis and it may be inappropriate to 'escalate treatment'. This is, as always, an issue that requires careful consideration and discussion with senior colleagues. The factors to be considered and the approach to be taken are very similar to those discussed in Section 1.10, p. 37, acute on chronic respiratory failure. (See also *General clinical issues*, Section 3.)

Principles of management of acute liver failure and hepatic encephalopathy:
• supportive measures
• treatment of metabolic abnormalities
• reduction of intestinal nitrogenous load
• treatment of coagulopathy
• treatment of underlying infection
• treatment of complications.

Acute alcohol withdrawal and delirium tremens

The following headings describe the important aspects of management of alcohol withdrawal and delirium tremens.

SUPPORTIVE MEASURES

• Obtain intravenous access and monitor urine output.
• Assess fluid balance and correct hypovolaemia.
• Monitor heart rate and rhythm and pulse oximetry.

SEDATION

• Chlordiazepoxide 10–50 mg qds is the treatment of choice if the patient can tolerate oral therapy.
• Give chlormethiazole i.v. if the patient is severely agitated and unable to tolerate oral therapy. This is administered as a 0.8% solution at an initial rate of 24–60 mg/min until shallow sleep is induced from which the patient can be easily roused. The rate is then reduced to the lowest possible to maintain shallow sleep and normal spontaneous respiration.

Chlormethiazole may cause respiratory depression. Patients must be closely monitored and full resuscitation facilities must be available.

TREATMENT OF SEIZURES

• Maintain the airway.
• Give O_2.
• Give diazepam 5–10 mg i.v.
• Consider starting a chlormethiazole infusion if seizures are not controlled by diazepam, but remember the risk of respiratory depression.
• Intubation and ventilation may be required for status epilepticus.

TREATMENT OF METABOLIC ABNORMALITIES

• Treat hypoglycaemia with glucose, but remember to give thiamine first.
• If severe hypophosphataemia is present, start potassium phosphate i.v. Monitor serum phosphate and calcium closely.
• Vitamin supplementation—as above.

Acute alcohol withdrawal may cause tremor and confusion after 8–24 h which usually settles after 48 h.
Delirium tremens is rare but can be fatal if untreated. Symptoms include tremor, confusion, visual hallucinations, fever and sweating. It usually occurs 3–4 days after stopping drinking.

See *Gastroenterology*, Sections 1.7, 1.8, 1.16, 2.9 and 2.10. O'Grady JG, Williams RS. Acute hepatic failure. In: Tinker J, Zapol WM, eds. *Care of the Critically Ill Patient*, 2nd edn. London: Springer Verlag, 1992: 609–620.

1.15 Renal failure, fluid overload and hyperkalaemia

Case history

A 30-year-old man with chronic renal failure and who is on regular haemodialysis is visiting the area and is brought to A&E because his friends are worried about him. He has been with them for a stag weekend and has been drinking for 12 h. He appears confused and is hyperventilating.

Clinical approach

The immediate priority is to detect and treat any life-threatening complications of renal failure.

Why is he breathing fast?

• Could he be in pulmonary oedema? Does he have metabolic acidosis?

- Give high-flow O_2, check pulse oximetry and measure arterial blood gases.

Does he have hyperkalaemia?

Get an immediate ECG. What are the features of hyperkalaemia? What is the emergency treatment? (See management, p. 53.)

Consider the differential diagnosis of his reduced conscious level

Could he:
- be nearly dead?
- be uraemic?
- have a head injury?
- be suffering from drug or alcohol intoxication?

Background information

Once resuscitation is underway, phone the patient's local dialysis centre. Two minutes talking to a renal physician or dialysis nurse who knows him will probably help enormously: 'Oh, you've got Eric have you … ?'

History of the presenting problem

This patient's state is probably due to excessive alcohol and fluid intake. Check:
- what and how much has he drunk?
- when did he last dialyse?

But think also about other precipitants of deterioration in those with renal failure:
- infection
- fluid loss, e.g. prolonged vomiting or diarrhoea
- drugs—including over-the-counter medications and street drugs.

And in this case:
- has he had a fall and banged his head?
- has he been in a fight?

Relevant past history

Information that is important includes:
- The underlying cause of his renal failure. Is it an ongoing problem, e.g. diabetes?
- What is his normal dialysis regimen?
- Has he had this sort of trouble in the past?
- Does he have any other major medical problems?

Examination

Immediate priorities are:
- Check airway, breathing, circulation.

- Is the patient well, ill, very ill or nearly dead? If he is nearly dead, call for ICU help immediately.
- Check GCS in anyone with impaired consciousness.
  Further examination should concentrate on assessment of fluid status and looking for evidence of causes of confusion.

Assessment of fluid status

Take careful note of the following:
- Respiratory rate—tachypnoea could indicate fluid overload or acidosis. But beware of a normal respiratory rate in someone who looks exhausted: this may mean that they are about to die (see Section 1.7, p. 27).
- Pulse rate and rhythm.
- Blood pressure—is this very high? It might be in a fluid-overloaded dialysis patient. But also check for postural hypotension (lying and sitting—a drop in pressure indicating intravascular volume depletion) and paradox (is there tamponade?).
- JVP—you must decide: is this high (could be very high) or low (could be very low)?
- Heart sounds—is there a gallop rhythm, indicating that the left ventricle is under strain, or a pericardial rub, probably uraemic in this context?
- Lung bases—are there crackles, suggesting pulmonary oedema in this case?
- Peripheral oedema—which is likely to indicate long-term fluid overload in a dialysis patient.

Other assessment

Check:
- Temperature—has he got a high fever, suggesting infection?
- Chest—does the patient have Kussmaul's breathing, indicating metabolic (probably uraemic) acidosis? Are there focal signs? These might indicate pneumonia, perhaps due to aspiration.
- Abdomen—has he got tenderness or guarding? Has there been an intra-abdominal catastrophe? Has he developed pancreatitis?
- Neurology—has he got neck stiffness, which might be due to meningitis or subarachnoid haemorrhage, or any focal signs, possibly (given the sudden onset of problems) indicating a stroke?
- Are there any signs of head injury?

Approach to investigations and management

Investigations

Electrocardiogram

A 12-lead ECG must be done immediately in any ill

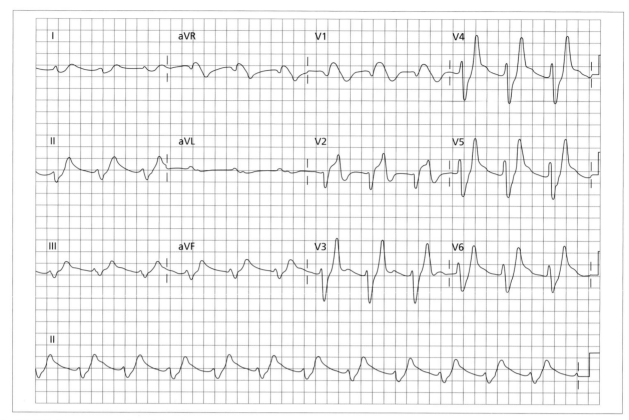

Fig. 32 ECG changes in severe hyperkalaemia.

patient, especially one known to have renal failure, to look for changes of hyperkalaemia (see Key point below and Fig. 32). Also look for evidence of myocardial ischaemia or pericarditis.

 Hyperkalaemia can kill suddenly and without warning. The following ECG changes occur sequentially as the serum potassium rises:
1 tall 'peaked' T waves
2 flattened P waves, prolonged P-R interval, wide QRS complexes
3 cardiac arrest—VF, VT, asystole.

Urgent treatment is required if there is any change more severe than T-wave peaking; take a specimen for measurement of the serum potassium, but do not wait for the result! It is not a triumph to be told that the serum potassium was 9.1 mmol/L just after the patient has arrested.

Blood tests and cultures

Check:
• Arterial blood gases—expect a partially compensated metabolic acidosis in a sick patient with renal failure. A normal $Pa\text{CO}_2$ would probably be worrying in this case, indicating that the patient is getting tired and losing respiratory compensation, in which case acidosis can worsen very rapidly with dire consequences.

• Urea and electrolytes, full blood count (raised white cell count may indicate infection) and blood cultures.
• Culture—swab from around dialysis access sites (indwelling neck lines, peritoneal dialysis catheters) if these look inflamed; peritoneal dialysis fluid (if applicable); urine (if the patient is not anuric).

Chest radiograph

Check for heart size (is there a pericardial effusion?), pulmonary oedema and infection.

Management

 Indications for urgent dialysis in renal failure

• Persistent hyperkalaemia.
• Refractory pulmonary oedema.
• Severe metabolic acidosis.
• Symptomatic uraemia, e.g. altered mental status, fits, asterixis, pericarditis.

Correction of life-threatening complications obviously takes priority:
• hyperkalaemia
• severe fluid overload
• severe metabolic acidosis.

Hyperkalaemia

If there are ECG changes more severe than tenting of the T waves (Fig. 32), then treatment must be immediate to prevent cardiac arrest.
• Give 10 mL 10% calcium gluconate i.v.—this does not lower potassium level but reduces myocardial excitability. Its effect is instant: the ECG 'improves' in front of your eyes.

Then:
• Give 50 mL 50% dextrose with 10 U short-acting insulin (e.g. Actrapid) over 15–30 min. This shifts potassium into the intracellular compartment. It should not cause hypoglycaemia, but check BM stix if in any doubt. Serum potassium falls by 1–2 mmol/L over 20–30 min.

And/or:
• Give 5–10 mg nebulized salbutamol, which activates the intracellular adenylate cyclase system inducing a shift of potassium into the intracellular compartment. Serum potassium falls by 1–2 mmol/L over 20–30 min.

Another option if the patient has metabolic acidosis, is to consider giving 1 mmol/kg 8.4% bicarbonate through a central line over 15–30 min. This is effective in reducing serum potassium, but its use should usually be restricted to those with severe acidosis that requires immediate treatment in its own right because of potential adverse effects. These include fluid overload/pulmonary oedema, hypernatraemia and hyperosmolarity. Remember also that 8.4% sodium bicarbonate should never be given through a peripheral line. It is extremely irritant and can cause nasty chemical burns if it gets into the tissues.

Do not forget to contact the local renal unit to arrange dialysis urgently! Calcium, dextrose/insulin, salbutamol (and bicarbonate) are holding measures only, reducing plasma potassium for 4–6 h only (if nothing else changes). This patient, a regular dialysis patient, will certainly need urgent dialysis if he is hyperkalaemic, as will most patients with severe hyperkalaemia in the context of acute renal failure, the exceptions being those whose renal function improves rapidly, e.g. those who become polyuric after relief of acute obstruction.

Oral and rectal ion exchange resins, which increase gut excretion of potassium, can be used to take the 'edge' off hyperkalaemia, but they are not an emergency treatment for a high serum potassium as they take 24 h to work.

Treatment of severe hyperkalaemia

- Give calcium gluconate i.v.
- Give insulin/dextrose i.v. or nebulized salbutamol.
- Arrange dialysis.
- Measure serum potassium frequently to monitor response to treatment.

Severe fluid overload

Prompt treatment is essential. In this man, who is a dialysis patient:
• sit the patient up
• give high-flow O_2
• use only minimal fluid when administering parenteral drugs
• start nitrates i.v., e.g. glyceryl trinitrate infusion 2–20 mL/h, titrated to as high a dose as the blood pressure will allow
• arrange urgent dialysis/ultrafiltration
• consider venesection of 1 U of blood if *in extremis*.

In a patient with acute renal failure who is overloaded it is also worth trying an intravenous infusion of furosemide (frusemide), 250 mg over 1 h. Up to 1 g of the drug can be given in this way over 24 h but with a rate not exceeding 4 mg/min.

Fluid overload and central lines

A central line may be necessary for treatment, e.g. dialysis access, but:
• do not lie the patient down to put one in—they are likely to arrest (Experienced operators may insert an internal jugular line with the patient lying at 45°.)
• do not use the subclavian vein—the patient will not tolerate a pneumothorax
• use the femoral vein.

Severe metabolic acidosis

If acidosis is sufficiently severe to be causing haemodynamic compromise in its own right (difficult to judge, but possible with pH <7.0), then:
• give 1 mmol/kg 8.4% bicarbonate through a central line over 15–30 min
• arrange for urgent dialysis.

Other aspects

It is likely that this patient is suffering from the effects of missed dialysis combined with fluid and alcohol challenge, and that he will improve with dialysis treatment. If any other diagnoses declare themselves, e.g. sepsis, they will require specific treatment on their merits.

See *Nephrology*, Sections 1.6 and 2.2.
Brady HR, Singer GG. Acute renal failure. *Lancet* 1995; 346: 1533–1540.
Harper J. Acute renal failure in CPD. *J Int Med* June 2000 Rila Publications. (contains a clear description of the treatment of hyperkalaemia).
Kemper MJ, Harps E, Muller-Wiefel DE. Hyperkalaemia: therapeutic options in acute and chronic renal failure. *Clin Nephrol* 1996; 46: 67–69.

1.16 Diabetic ketoacidosis

Case history

A 22-year-old student is brought to A&E by her boyfriend who has found her unwell and drowsy. He tells you that she has diabetes and has not been to lectures for 2 days as she has been vomiting. Her last BM stix reading was over 22 mmol/L.

Clinical approach

Diabetic ketoacidosis (DKA) should be considered in any insulin-dependent diabetic who becomes acutely unwell. The patient may be grossly dehydrated and acidotic. If this is left untreated, coma and death may ensue.

The priorities of emergency management are to confirm the diagnosis, treat dehydration and metabolic disturbance and identify precipitating factors, e.g. infection or any other acute intercurrent illness.

The differential diagnosis of altered conscious level, hyperglycaemia and/or acidosis in a diabetic patient is shown in Table 13.

History of the presenting problem

If the patient is unwell, take the history at the same time as gaining venous access and repeating the check of the BM stix measurement of glucose. Discover:
- Duration of symptoms.
- Current insulin regimen and compliance—poor compliance is a common cause of DKA.

Attempt to identify a precipitating cause and ask specifically about:
- Dysuria.
- Cough.
- Other sources of infection—including foot ulcers, dental abscesses and skin infections.
- Chest pain—not likely in this young woman, but remember that in middle-aged and older diabetics myocardial infarction is often silent.

Regarding the previous history, enquire about:

- Duration of diabetes.
- Complications of the disease—macrovascular (ischaemic heart disease, cerebrovascular disease and peripheral vascular disease) and microvascular (neuropathy, nephropathy and retinopathy).
- Earlier episodes of DKA or of hypoglycaemia.

DKA can be the first presentation of insulin-dependent diabetes.
It must be considered in any patient with a history of weight loss, polyuria, polydipsia, unexplained dehydration or acidosis.

Examination

What does the patient look like?—well, ill, very ill or nearly dead? The pace of action is dictated by this. The requirement is to assess fluid status and look for evidence of a precipitating factor.
- Check airway, breathing, circulation.
- Are they drowsy and confused?—check GCS.
- Is breathing acidotic (Kussmaul's respiration)?
- Do they smell of ketones?

Assessment of fluid status

Are they haemodynamically compromised? Check:
- Pulse rate.
- Blood pressure—lying and sitting. A recumbent blood pressure of 100/50 could be normal in this patient, but if the systolic falls to 70 when you sit her up, you know that she has substantial intravascular volume depletion.
- JVP—likely to be very low.

Note that interstitial and intracellular fluid will also be depleted, as well as intravascular. This will manifest itself as dry mucous membranes and reduced skin turgor, findings that would clearly be significant in this woman, but much harder to interpret in an elderly patient.

Other aspects

Check:
- Temperature—pyrexia usually indicates the presence of infection, but the patient may have septic shock even if apyrexial.

Altered conscious level	Hyperglycaemia	Acidosis (high anion gap)
DKA	DKA	DKA
HONC	HONC	Lactic acidosis (may occur with hyperglycaemia in HONC, or metformin therapy)
Hypoglycaemia (see Section 1.17, p. 57)	Sepsis (increased insulin resistance)	Uraemia
Another cause of coma (see Section 1.26, p. 75)		Salicylate poisoning (may have ↑ or ↓ glucose)

Table 13 Differential diagnoses to consider in unwell diabetic patients.

DKA, diabetic ketoacidosis; HONC, hyperosmolar non-ketotic diabetic coma.

- Chest—what is the respiratory rate? Look for signs of a chest infection.
- Abdomen—is there abdominal tenderness, silent bowel sounds or pain in the renal angles? Has an intraabdominal event triggered the DKA? Do not forget rectal examination: you will not see a perianal abscess unless you look.
- Feet—take the shoes off: are there any ulcers?
- Skin—are there any nasty spots or boils?

Diabetic ketoacidosis and the abdomen

- DKA may masquerade as an acute abdomen.
- Serum amylase may be high in the absence of pancreatitis.
- Abdominal emergencies precipitate DKA, especially in older patients.
- Be careful—if in doubt seek a senior surgical opinion.

Approach to investigations and management

Diabetic ketoacidosis is confirmed by the presence of hyperglycaemia, a low bicarbonate (<15 mmol/L and low pH <7.30) with ketonaemia or moderate/severe ketonuria. Check immediately:
- BM stix
- arterial blood gases
- urine with Ketostix.

Investigations

Blood tests

- Check serum glucose, U & Es, FBC and blood cultures.
- Have a low threshold for measuring cardiac enzymes.

In DKA:
- The serum potassium is high—but total body potassium is very depleted
- The white cell count may be high in the absence of infection.

Urine tests

Ketones will be moderately or strongly positive on Ketostix testing in DKA, but remember that ketonuria is normal after a period of starvation. Send urine for microscopy, culture and sensitivity.

Electrocardiograph

An ECG is essential in order to exclude myocardial infarction which is a common precipitant of DKA, although this is very unlikely in a 20-year-old woman.

Chest radiograph

Look specifically for evidence of infection and also for air under the diaphragms. Perforation of an abdominal viscus can be remarkably silent in the diabetic.

Management

Diabetic ketoacidosis

Priorities of management in a patient with DKA are:
- Correction of hypovolaemia.
- Correction of electrolyte imbalance.
- Correction of hyperglycaemia.
- Restoration of acid–base balance.
- Emptying the stomach.
- Treatment of any underlying cause.
- Prophylaxis against venous thromboembolism.

REPLACEMENT OF FLUID AND ELECTROLYTE LOSSES

Patients with DKA are severely dehydrated and very depleted of total body sodium and potassium. Fluid replacement is the priority in management. If hypovolaemic shock is present, colloid should be given initially, as described in Section 1.11, p. 39. Most patients do not require this and should be given 0.9% saline (normal saline) as shown in Table 14.

Diabetic ketoacidosis leads to a negative potassium balance through osmotic diuresis and acidaemia. In the first few hours of treatment with rehydration and insulin there will be a rapid decline in plasma potassium concentration due to re-entry of the ion into cells. Potassium must therefore be replaced as part of the fluid regimen after the first litre of normal saline has been delivered (Table 15). Monitor potassium levels closely throughout treatment.

Table 14 Fluid replacement in diabetic ketoacidosis.

1 L 0.9% saline over 30 min then:
1 L 0.9% saline + K+ (Table 15) over 1 h then:
1 L 0.9% saline + K+ over 2 h then:
1 L 0.9% saline + K+ 4-hourly until rehydrated

When blood glucose <15 mmol/L change fluid to 5% dextrose and continue insulin infusion

Table 15 Potassium replacement in diabetic ketoacidosis.

Plasma potassium (mmol/L)	Potassium (mmol) to add to each litre
<3	40
<4	30
<5	20

• Monitor potassium at least every few hours initially to avoid hypokalaemia (or hyperkalaemia if replacement is too enthusiastic).
• Administer less potassium in patients with renal impairment or oliguria.

CORRECTION OF HYPERGLYCAEMIA

Insulin therapy reverses ketogenesis, lowers blood sugar and therefore stops osmotic diuresis.

Commence an intravenous sliding scale of insulin by adding 50 units of Actrapid to 50 mL of normal saline and setting the rate of infusion as shown in Table 16. Monitor blood sugar hourly while the infusion is running.

Continue the insulin infusion after normoglycaemia has been achieved and give intravenous dextrose (5% or 10% as necessary) instead of saline in order to inhibit ketogenesis until the serum and urine are clear of ketones and the metabolic acidosis has been corrected.

RESTORATION OF ACID–BASE BALANCE

If there is adequate renal function and tissue perfusion, restoration of normovolaemia will rapidly reverse the lactate component of metabolic acidosis. Insulin reverses ketogenesis and also causes oxidation of existing ketones, resulting in endogenous bicarbonate production.

The use of bicarbonate in the treatment of DKA is controversial, although it should be considered if the acidaemia is extreme (pH <7.0) and thought to be causing

Table 16 Sliding scale for treatment of DKA.

BM measured hourly	Insulin rate (units/h)
<4	0.5
4–7.0	1
7.1–11	2
11.1–15	3
15.1–19	4
19.1–24	5
>24	6

DKA, diabetic ketoacidosis.

circulatory compromise in its own right (see Section 1.15, p. 53).

Bicarbonate administration in DKA should be considered only in extreme acidosis. It may cause:
• Exacerbation of hypokalaemia.
• Paradoxical intracellular acidosis due to increased CO_2 production.
• Shift of the O_2 dissociation curve to the left.
• Late alkalosis.

EMPTY THE STOMACH

A drowsy diabetic with DKA may have gastroparesis and several litres of acid stomach contents waiting to be vomited: aspiration can be fatal. Pass a nasogastric tube and empty the stomach. If there is nothing there, pull it out.

TREAT THE UNDERLYING CAUSE OF DKA

Infection is a common precipitant of DKA and the diabetic may not manifest the classical signs of toxicity when infection is present. Commence broad-spectrum antibiotics empirically after taking cultures of blood and urine, working on the premise that infection is the cause until proved otherwise. Localized infection, e.g. foot ulcer, may require 'surgical attention'.

Exclude myocardial infarction and other cardiovascular catastrophes (including PE) regardless of the age of the patient.

PROPHYLAXIS AGAINST VENOUS THROMBOEMBOLISM

An immobile dehydrated patient is at high risk of venous thromboembolism: prescribe prophylactic low molecular weight heparin.

MANAGEMENT OF COMPLICATIONS

Monitor closely for signs of complications of treatment (Table 17).

Table 17 Complications of treatment of DKA.

Complication	Cause	Treatment
Hypoglycaemia	Not enough dextrose given	Change intravenous fluid to 5% dextrose when BM >15
Hypokalaemia	Not enough K⁺ given	Replace K⁺ with fluid (Table 15)
Cerebral oedema	Rapid decrease in extracellular osmolality	Consider intravenous mannitol
ARDS	? Excessive crystalloid infusion	Respiratory support as needed
Hypophosphataemia	Phosphate moves intracellularly with potassium	Replace if levels <0.5 mmol/L
Hyperchloraemic acidosis	Excessive sodium chloride administration. Intracellular shift of bicarbonate	No treatment required. Will correct by enhanced renal excretion

ARDS, acute respiratory distress syndrome; DKA, diabetic ketoacidosis.

Cerebral oedema is a rare but potentially fatal complication of DKA or its treatment. Suspect it if the patient complains of a headache or is drowsy or confused. Seek senior help. Intensive care will be necessary.

Hyperosmolar non-ketotic diabetic coma

Hyperosmolar non-ketotic diabetic coma (HONC) must be considered in any patient with severe hyperglycaemia. Like DKA it is a metabolic emergency and the mortality rate is high. It is typically seen in elderly patients with non-insulin-dependent diabetes and is commonly precipitated by intercurrent illness. Various medications (e.g. thiazide diuretics, steroids) and consumption of glucose-rich fluid, e.g. Lucozade, can also precipitate it. Patients are not (by definition) ketoacidotic, but may be acidotic due to lactate accumulation as a result of poor tissue perfusion with or without renal failure. The approach to investigations and management is similar to that for DKA but there are additional points to bear in mind.

DIAGNOSIS

Look for the following:
• Plasma osmolality is >350 mOsml/kg. This is calculated by:

$2 \times [(Na^+ + K^+) + Urea + Glucose]$(with Na^+, K^+, Urea and Glucose all measured in mool/l)

• Glucose is usually >40 mmol/L.
• There may be marked hypernatraemia.
• Dehydration tends to be severe, causing a disproportionately raised plasma urea.
• Arterial blood gases are usually relatively normal with pH >7.3 (unless there is lactate accumulation).

TREATMENT

The use of hypotonic fluid for rehydration is controversial, the fear being that too rapid reduction of hypernatraemia may be deleterious, resulting in neurological damage (perhaps central pontine myelinolysis—although evidence is incomplete) and death.

The safest approach is to use 0.9% (normal) saline initially to restore blood pressure and urine flow and then to change to 0.45% saline if plasma Na^+ is still >150 mmol/L to replace the free water deficit.

Insulin requirements tend to be low, therefore start at a lower dose of insulin and monitor BM stix closely to avoid hypoglycaemia.

Patients with HONC are particularly prone to thromboembolism: anticoagulate with low-molecular-weight heparin as routine.

Why did it happen?

> To have one episode of diabetic ketoacidosis may be described as misfortune. To have two smacks of carelessness.

Diabetics do not develop DKA or HONC overnight. The metabolic picture builds up over several days. In those known to have diabetes, these dangerous conditions are almost invariably avoidable, and when a patient has recovered from an episode they should not leave hospital without advice about how to avoid another. They should be told:
• If you get ill, you are likely to need more insulin rather than less.
• If you get ill, check your blood sugar at least four times a day.
• If the sugar is going up and you do not know what to do—call for help.

Bell DSH, Alele J. Diabetic ketoacidosis. Why early detection and treatment are crucial. *Postgrad Med* 1997; 101: 193–204.
Kitabchi AE, Wall BM. Diabetic ketoacidosis. *Med Clin North Am* 1995; 79: 9–37.
Lorber D. Nonketotic hypertonicity in diabetes mellitus. *Med Clin North Am* 1995; 79: 39–52.

1.17 Hypoglycaemia

Case history

A 70-year-old woman with non-insulin-dependent diabetes is brought to A&E by ambulance after being found unconscious on the kitchen floor by her home-help. During transfer to hospital she had a generalized seizure and on arrival in the emergency room she is unresponsive to pain.

Clinical approach

Your first priority in any unconscious patient is ABC (airway, breathing, circulation). Check she is maintaining her own airway and give O_2.

Obtain venous access and do a BM immediately (Fig. 33). In this case hypoglycaemia was confirmed on BM stix (1.1 mmol/L) and intravenous sugar (50 mL of 50% dextrose injected into a large vein to minimize the risk of thrombophlebitis) was given immediately. Blood was taken to be sent for a laboratory glucose, but she was treated without waiting for the result. Urgent treatment is vital if permanent cerebral damage is to be avoided.

Table 18 descibes the differential diagnosis of spontaneous hypoglycaemia. The finding of profound

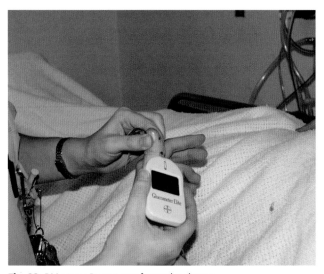

Fig. 33 BM meter. Do not ever forget the glucose.

Table 18 Causes of hypoglycaemia.

Diabetic patients	Non-diabetic patients
Insulin	Concealed insulin administration
Oral hypoglycaemics (especially longer-acting sulphonylureas)	Drugs (e.g. oral hypoglycaemics, quinine, pentamidine)
Excessive alcohol intake	Salicylate overdose
Excessive exercise	Excessive alcohol (especially chronic alcoholics with liver disease)
	Sepsis
	Insulinoma
	Retroperitoneal sarcoma
	Hypopituitarism
	Adrenocortical insufficiency
	Myxoedema
	Liver failure

hypoglycaemia was sufficient to explain coma, meaning that a wider differential diagnosis of coma (see Section 1.26, p. 75) did not have to be entertained immediately.

Priorities in an unconscious patient

- Airway.
- Breathing.
- Circulation.
- Do not ever forget the glucose.

History of the presenting problem

Most patients with hypoglycaemia will not be able to give a history. While they are being treated try to obtain relevant information from relatives or friends. Enquire about:
- History of diabetes and current treatment. Has it been changed recently?
- Complications of diabetes—hypoglycaemia is more common in diabetic nephropathy.
- Other drug treatment.
- Possible precipitating cause, e.g. alcohol intake.

Examination

Clinical examination is undertaken at the same time that treatment is initiated. Look specifically for the following:
- Check GCS—so that you know if she's getting better or worse when you repeat it in a few minutes.
- If collapsed—is there evidence of injury?
- If found on the floor—are there signs of pressure area damage? If there are, think of rhabdomyolysis (see *Nephrology*, Section 1.17).
- If there has been a fit—check the mouth and tongue for damage.

Once the patient has responded to treatment, perform a full neurological examination. In cases of severe, prolonged hypoglycaemia neurological deficit may persist for days or weeks, and sometimes permanently, despite correction of the blood sugar.

Approach to investigations and management

Investigations

Blood tests

- Blood should be drawn for tests before dextrose is given if at all possible (but do not delay treatment).
- Check blood glucose, U & Es and LFTs.
- In non-diabetics save serum for insulin levels and C-peptide.
- Check a salicylate level if there is any suspicion of overdose.

Management

This patient had already been given 50 mL of 50% dextrose i.v. and a prompt response was obtained. If intravenous access is impossible, give 1 mg glucagon intramuscularly, but remember that glucagon will not work if hypoglycaemia is due to alcohol.

Remember that the half-lives of oral hypoglycaemic agents and medium- and long-acting insulin preparations are longer than that of glucose. The patient should not be discharged the moment that they become conscious. Give a sugary drink and something to eat to prevent recurrent hypoglycaemia and monitor for at least a few hours. If hypoglycaemia recurs start an infusion of 10% dextrose aiming to maintain blood glucose at 5–10 mmol/L.

Hypoglycaemia in the 'down and out'

If there is a history of chronic alcohol intake or malnourishment give thiamine i.v. before glucose to avoid precipitating Wernicke's encephalopathy.

Hypoglycaemic coma

If the patient does not wake up within 15 min of treatment repeat the BM and consider the possibility of additional pathology, e.g. head injury or drug overdose.

Why did it happen?

Hypoglycaemia strikes some diabetics out of the blue, but most have some warning. Before the patient is discharged, talk through with them what (if anything) they remember of events before their admission. Impress upon them that hypoglycaemia is serious—it can be fatal. Tell them that if they get the same feelings again, they must check their blood sugar, and that they must have some sugar available to take at all times. With the patient's permission, it is also prudent to offer advice and instruction on how to recognize and handle hypoglycaemia to any of their family and friends that are available.

See *Endocrinology*, Section 1.4.

1.18 Hypercalcaemia and hyponatraemia

Case history

A 70-year-old man is brought to A&E by his daughter who says he has become increasingly confused and unwell over the past few days. She tells you he was diagnosed as having 'lung cancer' several months ago but has not received any specific treatment. He appears drowsy and disorientated.

Clinical approach

In any patient with malignancy who presents acutely unwell it is important to consider whether they have a metabolic cause for their symptoms that requires urgent treatment. The most important of these are hypercalcaemia and hyponatraemia.

The cause of the deterioration may be determined by a targeted history and examination followed by relevant investigations, but immediate priorities are:
• Give the patient O_2, check oximetry and put them on a cardiac monitor.
• Are they cardiovascularly stable? Obtain venous access.
• Consider the differential diagnosis of confusion and drowsiness in someone with known malignancy (Table 19).

Table 19 Common causes of confusion or drowsiness in a patient with malignancy.

Metabolic (hypercalcaemia, hyponatraemia, hypoglycaemia)
Hypoxia (primary lung tumours, pulmonary metastases, pleural effusion, pulmonary emboli)
Cerebral metastases
Encephalopathy (non-metastatic manifestation of bronchial carcinoma)
Drugs (e.g. opiates)
Infection

History of the presenting problem

The patient is unlikely to be able to give a complete and lucid history. Check his Abbreviated Mental Test score (see *Medicine for the elderly*, Sections 1.2 and 3.2) to establish a base-line, ask him simple questions and obtain as many details as possible from his daughter.

Ask specifically about symptoms of hypercalcaemia:
• abdominal pain
• nausea and vomiting
• constipation
• weight loss
• thirst and polyuria.

Ask about symptoms and causes of hyponatraemia:
• anorexia and nausea
• muscle cramps
• neurological symptoms—dizziness, light-headedness
• drug history—diuretics, thiazides particularly, may cause severe hyponatraemia.

Note that the symptoms of hypercalcaemia and hyponatraemia are non-specific. In many cases they can only be attributed to the electrolyte disturbance in retrospect if they improve with correction of the abnormality.

Ask about symptoms that might indicate other causes of confusion or drowsiness in this patient:
• headache—cerebral metastases
• pain—opiate toxicity
• fevers, sweats—infection.

Examination

Look at the general condition of the patient, check vital signs and then concentrate on the points discussed below.

Assessment of fluid status

Assess:
• Intravascular volume—check pulse, blood pressure (lying and sitting) and JVP.
• Interstitial/cellular fluid volume—check skin turgor, mucous membranes and peripheral oedema.

Is there evidence of malignancy?

Look for:
- cachexia
- lymphadenopathy
- hepatomegaly.

And thinking particularly of lung cancer:
- signs in the chest
- clubbing
- Horner's syndrome (Fig. 34)
- hypertrophic pulmonary osteoarthropathy (Fig. 35).

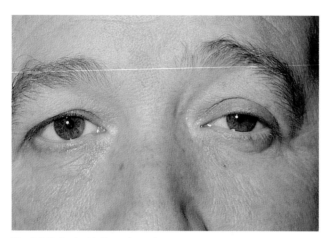

Fig. 34 Patient with Horner's syndrome.

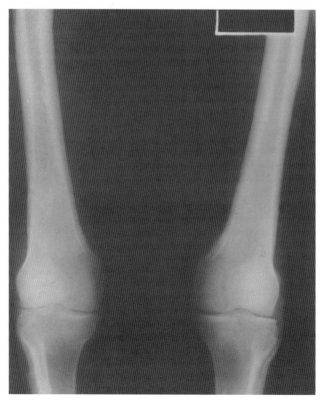

Fig. 35 Hypertrophic pulmonary osteoarthropathy.

Are there clues to other specific causes of confusion and drowsiness?

Check:
- Pupils and respiratory rate—small pupils and low respiratory rate probably mean opiate toxicity. If present, give naloxone (see Section 1.26, p. 75).
- Fundi—papilloedema would indicate raised intracranial pressure and almost certainly cerebral metastases in this man.
- Neurological examination—clear focal signs suggest a focal brain lesion, e.g. metastases, rather than something 'metabolic'.

Approach to investigations and management

Investigations

Blood tests

- Check U & Es, calcium, phosphate, magnesium, LFTs and FBC.
- Take blood cultures.
- Measure arterial blood gases.

Interpretation of serum calcium concentration

Free (ionized) plasma calcium is dependent on plasma albumin:

Corrected calcium = measured calcium + [40 − serum albumin (g/L)] × 0.02

Electrocardiogram

This test should be performed in anyone who is acutely and inexplicably unwell. It could show evidence of silent myocardial infarction, but look specifically for brady-arrythmias and a short Q-T interval that may be associated with hypercalcaemia.

Chest radiograph

Look for confirmation of lung malignancy (Fig. 36) and also for bony secondaries/rib fractures and for pneumonia.

Management

Emergency management

HYPERCALCAEMIA

Urgent treatment of hypercalcaemia is needed if there is:
- a reduced conscious level
- confusion

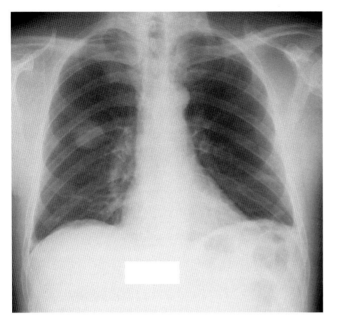

Fig. 36 Chest radiograph showing bronchogenic carcinoma.

- haemodynamic disturbance: intravascular volume depletion or gross dehydration.

> **Principles of emergency management of hypercalcaemia**
>
> - Increase urinary excretion of calcium by rehydration.
> - Inhibit bone resorption by bisphosphonate therapy.

Rehydration
The first aspect of emergency management should be rehydration with intravenous saline:
- If there is intravascular volume depletion give 0.9% (normal) saline rapidly until replete (see Section 1.11, p. 38).
- Then give 0.9% (normal) saline i.v. at a rate of around 4 L in 24 h. Insert a urinary catheter to monitor urine output. Stop infusion before fluid overload has been induced if the patient does not pass a good volume of urine! Consider giving furosemide (frusemide) 40–80 mg i.v. to encourage urine output if this is sluggish.
- Monitor calcium level, and also potassium and magnesium, which may fall rapidly with rehydration. Replace as necessary.

Bisphosphonate therapy
Disodium pamidronate is the drug of first choice for hypercalcaemia associated with malignancy: 15–60 mg i.v. is the standard dose, given slowly (over 4–6 h) into a large vein.

Glucocorticoids
Glucocorticoids are the treatment of choice for hypercalcaemia caused by vitamin D toxicity, sarcoidosis or myeloma. Give hydrocortisone 200 mg i.v. or prednisolone 40–60 mg orally.

> **Effect of steroids on hypercalcaemia**
>
> The main mechanism of action of steroids is to decrease 1,25-dihydroxyvitamin D levels by inhibiting inflammatory cell proliferation within granulomatous tissue and haematological malignancies. Although they also decrease intestinal calcium absorption and increase urinary calcium excretion, this occurs relatively slowly and they are of limited use in hypercalcaemia due to other causes.

HYPONATRAEMIA

> **Critical things to know about hyponatraemia**
>
> - Patients with hyponatraemia have too much water on board: they are almost never short of sodium.
> - Hyponatraemia that has developed slowly is often well tolerated and should be corrected slowly, usually with water restriction alone.
> - Hyponatraemia that has developed quickly is much rarer and often iatrogenic. It is much more likely to cause symptoms and to require rapid correction with hypertonic saline.
> - Correction of hyponatraemia that is too rapid and which 'overshoots' can be associated with dire neurological consequences (central pontine myelinolysis).

Asymptomatic
The emphasis in asymptomatic hyponatraemia is on treating the underlying disturbance (Table 20). Clinical assessment of the patient's fluid status is critical to making the correct diagnosis and thereby giving the correct treatment.

Table 20 Causes of hyponatraemia.

Decreased extracellular volume	Normal/mildly increased extracellular volume	Markedly increased extracellular volume
Gastrointestinal fluid losses (diarrhoea and vomiting with hypotonic fluid replacement)	SIAD (e.g. CNS disorders, malignancy, pulmonary disorders)	Congestive cardiac failure
Renal fluid losses (adrenocorticoid deficiency, diuretics, salt-losing nephropathies)	Drugs (e.g. carbamazepine, clofibrate, cyclophosphamide, chlorpropamide, thiazides, vasopressin, oxytocin, tricyclic antidepressants)	Cirrhosis with ascites
Burns	Severe hypothyroidism	Nephrotic syndrome
	Psychogenic polydipsia	Chronic renal failure

SIAD, syndrome of inappropriate antidiuresis.

Water restriction (1 L/day) should always allow the serum sodium concentration to rise but it can be difficult for patients to tolerate and for nurses to enforce. Give the allocation in aliquots throughout the day; give it as ice cubes to suck; allow the patient swabs to keep their mouth moist, or to suck boiled sweets.

Symptomatic

Urgent treatment is only required if there are severe neurological effects, e.g. fitting. Aside from treating the underlying cause:
• Start hypertonic (1.8%) saline at a rate of 50 ml/h until serum sodium >125 mmol/L. Aim to increase serum sodium concentration by around 1–2 mmol/h. If the concentration increases faster than this change to normal (0.9%) saline.
• Measure U & Es hourly initially to avoid too rapid correction of serum sodium: never aim to increase this by more than 12 mmol/L/day.
• When serum sodium >125 mmol/L stop intravenous saline and institute water restriction.
• In patients with the syndrome of inappropriate antidiuresis (SIAD) consider demeclocycline 150 mg every 6 hours.

Is hyponatraemia the cause of the patient's problems? Hyponatraemia alone will only cause neurological symptoms when the concentration is <120 mmol/L. If plasma sodium concentration is higher than this in a comatose patient, consider other causes of coma.

Severe hyponatraemia

The commonest cause of this is iatrogenic: postoperative infusion of excessive volumes of 5% dextrose solution.

Non-osmotic stimuli for antidiuretic hormone (ADH) release include haemorrhage, nausea, pain and anaesthesia. All of these can be present immediately after operations, leading to enormously high levels of ADH and inability to excrete water. If a stupid doctor prescribes large quantities of 5% dextrose the consequences can be dire. Do not do it!

How far do I go?

If this patient deteriorates, what should you do?

If the diagnosis of malignant disease is certain, then you need to decide, with expert advice from oncological colleagues, what the likely prognosis is. If it is bleak, then transfer to ICU or attempts to perform cardiac resuscitation would almost certainly be futile, unkind and inappropriate. These are issues that will need to be discussed with his daughter and (depending on his condition) with the patient himself. For suggestions on how to approach these matters, see *General clinical issues*, Section 3.

See *Pain relief and palliative care*, Section 1.4; *Endocrinology*, Sections 1.1 and 1.2.
Edelson GW, Kleerekoper M. Hypercalcaemic crisis. *Med Clin North Am* 1995; 79: 79–92.
Mulloy AL, Caruana RJ. Hyponatraemic emergencies. *Med Clin North Am* 1995; 79: 155–168.

1.19 Metabolic acidosis

Case history

A 23-year-old female student from the local university is admitted via A&E one Saturday night. She lives in halls of residence on her own and has been discovered semi-conscious by a student neighbour. No medical records are available and she is unaccompanied in the ambulance.

The referral note describes her as 'a quiet, introverted girl who has few friends' and there is a strong suggestion that she has lost weight over the preceding few weeks. When you see her, she is hyperventilating and has a GCS of 10/15 (E:3, V:3, M:4). She is covered in vomit.

Clinical approach

Your first priorities are:
• Airway, breathing, circulation—as always!
• Check BM stix—give 50% dextrose 50 mL i.v. if hypoglycaemia. If blood sugar is very high then the working diagnosis becomes DKA (see Section 1.16, p. 54).
• Are pupils constricted and respiratory rate slow? If they are, working diagnosis is opiate toxicity. Give naloxone 0.4 mg i.v.
• Ensure adequate venous access.
Then proceed as shown below.

History of the presenting problem

She cannot give an account, but has anyone come up to A&E with her? If so, ask the following questions that might lead to a diagnosis:
• Does she have any medical problems?—ask specifically about diabetes and epilepsy.
• When did you last see her?
• Do you know if she has complained of being unwell over the last few days?
• Has this sort of thing happened before?
• Do you know if she has drunk a lot of alcohol?
• Is there any suggestion that she may have taken an overdose?
• Were tablets or bottles found at the scene?
• Has a suicide note been discovered?

Examination

Thorough general and neurological examinations are required, taking particular note of the following:
• vital signs—temperature, pulse, blood pressure, respiratory rate and pulse oximetry
• does she smell of alcohol?
• has she aspirated?
• are there lateralizing neurological signs? These would make a focal brain lesion more likely
• is there any evidence of meningitis? Exclude neck stiffness and other signs of meningism and search carefully for the tell-tale non-blanching petechiae of meningococcal septicaemia (see *Infectious diseases*, Section 1.14).

 The early rash of meningococcal septicaemia can be very unimpressive and often appears first in 'awkward' areas: buttocks, backs of the thighs and the flanks.

Approach to investigations and management

The examination gave a clue to the diagnosis: she was hyperventilating, which invokes the following possibilities:
• cardiorespiratory disease
• neurological pathology
• metabolic acidosis
• primary hyperventilation—but this seems vanishingly unlikely in this case and should be considered only after organic pathology has been excluded.

Investigations

The immediate priorities are shown below.

Arterial blood gases

These will confirm or exclude metabolic acidosis and are indicated as the first test in this case where there is abnormal respiration. The patient's arterial blood gas results, breathing air, were:
• PaO_2 13 kPa
• $PaCO_2$ 2.1 kPa
• pH   7.05
• Standard base excess   -17 mmol/L

This is the picture of severe metabolic acidosis with secondary (compensatory) hyperventilation. With this information, test immediately for the following common causes:
• Diabetic ketoacidosis. The blood sugar will be high and urinary and plasma ketones will be present (see Section 1.16, p. 54).

• Salicylate poisoning. The salicylate level will be high, this being the anion responsible for the acidosis (see Section 2.1, p. 86).
• Renal failure. What are the urea and creatinine?

If none of the above, is this lactic acidosis? The plasma lactate will be elevated (by definition). Possible causes include: compromised cardiac output for whatever reason, e.g. heart failure, PE or tamponade; liver failure—always consider paracetamol poisoning; and overwhelming sepsis.

WHAT IF THESE ARE NOT THE ANSWER?

Are there unusual anions around?—the presence of these, e.g. antifreeze, can be suspected from calculation of the anion gap. The number of positively and negatively charged ions in the blood must always be equal. If the concentrations of the commonly measured positively charged ions (sodium and potassium) are added together and subtracted from the concentrations of the commonly measured negatively charged ions (chloride and bicarbonate), then:

$$(Na^+ + K^+) - (Cl^- + HCO_3^-) \text{ normally equals } 10–18 \text{ mmol/L}$$

These 10–18 mmol/L—the 'anion gap'—are attributable to negatively charged proteins, phosphate, sulphate and some organic acids. If there is acidosis with a high anion gap, then there must be an unmeasured substance around.

Antifreeze can be measured in the blood. The specific antidote is alcohol.

After arterial blood gases, arrange the other investigations discussed below.

Blood tests

• Check full blood count, electrolytes, glucose, renal and liver function tests.
• Check toxicology screen, which should include urgent paracetamol and salicylate levels.
• Check serum bicarbonate and lactate if the answer is not apparent from previous test results.

Chest radiograph

The collapsed patient with a reduced level of consciousness commonly aspirates and appropriate antibiotics should be administered as soon as possible if there is evidence for this.

Electrocardiogram

Primary dysrhythmias, hypertrophic obstructive cardiomyopathy and anatomical abnormalities of the coronary arteries can all manifest as a cardiovascular catastrophe in the young adult with reduced conscious level and lactic acidosis as the presenting features.

Management

In this young woman, salicylate levels were diagnostic of overdose. She was treated as indicated in Section 2.1 (p. 86) and went on to make a full medical recovery. She was found to be suffering from profound depression and required inpatient psychiatric treatment, which was also successful, and she has since returned to her university studies.

Important points to remember

HEAD CT SCAN

Abnormal neurological signs or a reduced conscious level which cannot be explained on the basis of metabolic pathology are absolute indications for an urgent CT scan.

LUMBAR PUNCTURE

This is mandatory if meningitis, encephalitis or subarachnoid haemorrhage is suspected and a CT scan does not provide the diagnosis for coma.

The comatose patient who might have infection—shoot first, ask questions later.
Empirical treatment with antibiotics or acyclovir should be administered if meningitis or *Herpes simplex* encephalitis is suspected. Clinical deterioration can be rapid in either condition, even to the stage of rendering the patient unsalvageable. Specific treatment should not be delayed while either diagnosis is secured (see Section 1.26, p. 75).

See Sections 1.26, p. 75 and 2.1, p. 83; *Respiratory medicine*, Section 3.6.
Smithies M. Acid–base disturbances. In: Tinker J, Zapol WM, eds. *Care of the Critically Ill Patient*, 2nd edn. London: Springer-Verlag, 1992.

1.20 An endocrine crisis

Case history

A 28-year-old woman is brought to A&E by her husband after collapsing at home. She has been unwell for a while with weight loss, lethargy and dizziness. She is drowsy and complaining of abdominal discomfort and is found to be hypotensive by the nursing staff.

Clinical approach

Priorities, as always, are:
- Airway, breathing, circulation.
- High-flow O_2, monitor O_2 saturation and check arterial blood gases.
- Is she haemodynamically stable? Check pulse, blood pressure and JVP. Establish intravenous access and correct hypovolaemia if present (see Section 1.11, p. 38).
- Check the BM stix—rule out hypoglycaemia, always a priority in a drowsy patient.
- Check pupils (are they constricted?) and respiratory rate (is this slow?—could this be opiate overdose, another priority in someone who is drowsy?).

You are proceeding along the lines described in Sections 1.19 (p. 62) and 1.26 (p. 75), both of which deal with patients presenting with impaired consciousness. You find her blood pressure to be 80/50, and the lab rings up to say that her electrolytes are Na 128 mmol/L and K 5.6 mmol/L.
- What is the diagnosis?
- What parts of the history and examination should you now repeat?
- What is the treatment?
Read on for the answers.

The second clinical approach

Hypotension, hyponatraemia and hyperkalaemia are characteristic of Addison's disease. Unexplained weight loss, general symptoms of malaise and lethargy and abdominal discomfort are classical presenting features of this condition. The clinical approach is now to:
- repeat aspects of the history and examination that might support this diagnosis
- consider the causes of adrenocortical insufficiency (see *Endocrinology*, Section 2.2).
- determine what may have precipitated the crisis—infection and trauma being common examples.

History of the presenting problem

Ask about features of adrenal insufficiency:
- dizziness on standing: this may indicate postural hypotension
- nausea and vomiting
- abdominal pain
- non-specific symptoms such as weight loss, fatigue, weakness and myalgia

What might have precipitated the crisis? Any intercurrent illness?

Have there been symptoms of infection?

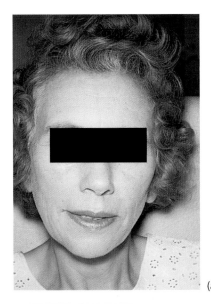

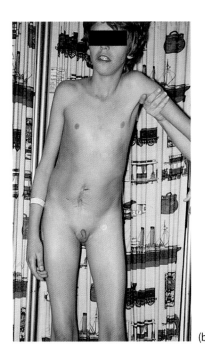

(a)

(b)

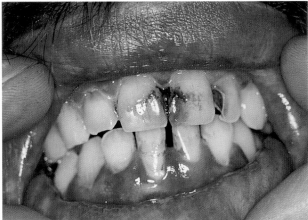

(c)

Fig. 37 Hyperpigmentation (a, b) and buccal pigmentation (c) in patients with Addison's disease. (From Axford J. *Medicine*. Oxford: Blackwell Science, 1996, with permission.)

What might be the cause of the Addison's disease? Ask about:
- previous endocrine/autoimmune disease
- a family history of endocrine/autoimmune disease
- drug history—has she taken steroids at any time in the past? These might have suppressed her adrenals and left her vulnerable to addisonian crisis with intercurrent stress
- history of tuberculosis
- flank pain—possibly indicating haemorrhagic adrenal infarction.

 To avoid precipitation of an addisonian crisis in patients who are on long-term corticosteroid treatment or who have known hypoadrenalism, give intravenous hydrocortisone if they present with an intercurrent illness or trauma.

Examination

You will obviously have concentrated on assessment of fluid status in a hypotensive patient, and have arranged resuscitation if intravascular volume is depleted (see Section 1.11, p. 38). You will have performed a thorough general examination, looking especially for indication of sepsis, but now:
- Is there pigmentation? Look specifically at the palmar creases and buccal mucosa (Fig. 37).
- Is there vitiligo, an association of autoimmune Addison's disease?

Approach to investigations and management

Investigations

The tests described in Section 1.19 (p. 63) will have been ordered, but now take a specimen to measure serum cortisol.

Typical findings in acute adrenal insufficiency:
- hyponatraemia
- hyperkalaemia
- hypoglycaemia.

Management

Emergency treatment of an addisonian crisis includes all of the following:
- Vigorous intravenous fluid replacement—give 0.9% (normal) saline rapidly until the JVP is normal.
- Glucocorticoid replacement—give hydrocortisone 200 mg i.v. stat and then 50–100 mg tds.
- Treatment of the precipitating cause—give empirical antibiotics if there is any suspicion of infection.
- Be aware of the risk of hypoglycaemia—monitor BM stix regularly: put up a 10% dextrose drip if necessary and run it at the rate necessary to keep glucose >5 mmol/L. Do not give more than is needed to do this, and avoid using 5% dextrose because it is more likely to exacerbate hyponatraemia.

In the patient who is not known to have Addison's disease, then the diagnosis can be confirmed by a short synacthen test. However, it is a bad mistake to delay treatment if the patient is unwell. Hydrocortisone can be switched to dexamethasone, which will not interfere with cortisol assay, to allow the test to be performed.

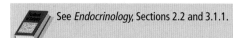 See *Endocrinology*, Sections 2.2 and 3.1.1.

1.21 Another endocrine crisis

Case history

A 45-year-old woman is brought to A&E by her daughter as she has become increasingly 'jittery' over the past few days. She has lost a lot of weight and has developed a marked tremor. Her daughter tells you that she is known to have 'a thyroid problem' but thinks she has recently stopped taking her usual tablets as she has become interested in homeopathic medicine.

Clinical approach

It is important to consider a thyrotoxic crisis in any patient who is known to have hyperthroidism and who is unwell. Mortality is high (up to 20–30% is reported). Urgent action is required:

Table 21 Precipitants of thyrotoxic crisis.

Infection
Withdrawal of antithyroid drug therapy
Radio-iodine treatment
Iodinated contrast dyes
Thyroid surgery
Childbirth
? Any intercurrent stress

- Give O_2 and attach a cardiac monitor.
- Is the patient cardiovascularly stable? Check pulse, blood pressure and venous pressure.
- Establish venous access.
- Monitor SaO_2 and measure arterial blood gases if <95%.
- Give specific treatment for thyrotoxic crisis on clinical suspicion; do not wait for the results of investigations.
- Treat any precipitating cause, if possible (Table 21). In this case withdrawal of antithyroid medication seems the obvious culprit, but always consider infection.

History of the presenting problem

There is usually, as in this case, a history of previous thyroid disease or of symptoms consistent with thyrotoxicosis that have been present for some time. Ask specifically about:
- weight loss
- palpitations
- heat intolerance
- sweating
- diarrhoea
- tremor
- anxiety/agitation/irritability
- possible precipitating causes (Table 21)
- a previous history or family history of endocrine/autoimmune disease.

Examination

In particular, concentrate on the following:
- Temperature—hyperpyrexia is a feature of thyrotoxic crisis and does not necessarily indicate infection.
- The skin is usually warm and moist.

Cardiovascular assessment

Look for signs of cardiovascular decompensation:
- tachycardia—in particular fast atrial fibrillation or supraventricular tachycardia
- cardiac failure—raised JVP, gallop rhythm, pulmonary oedema and peripheral oedema.

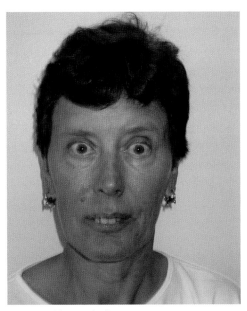

Fig. 38 A patient with Grave's disease.

The thyroid and related signs

Does the patient have signs of Grave's disease (Fig. 38)? Look for tremor, hyperkinesis, exophthalmos, lid lag and lid retraction.

Is there a goitre? If so, what are its characteristics (smooth, nodular, painful), and is there an associated bruit?

Does the patient have vitiligo, an association of auto-immune thyroid disease?

Approach to investigations and management

Thyrotoxic crisis:
• There are no laboratory criteria to diagnose thyrotoxic crisis.
• The levels of thyroid hormones are the same as in uncomplicated hyperthroidism.
• If the patient has a thyrotoxic crisis clinically, treatment should not be delayed while waiting for laboratory confirmation.

Investigations

The following are appropriate:
• Blood tests—check U & Es, FBC, glucose, thyroid function tests, LFTs and calcium. Send blood for culture.
• Electrocardiogram—look for atrial fibrillation and other dysrhythmias.
• Chest radiograph—look for evidence of pulmonary oedema or infection.

Management

Treatment

HYPERTHYROIDISM

• Give propylthiouracil 600 mg—1 g p.o./ng loading dose, then 200 mg qds. This blocks further synthesis of thyroid hormones and also inhibits peripheral T4 to T3 conversion.
• Carbimazole 20 mg 8-hourly may be used as an alternative to propylthiouracil but is less effective.
• Give Lugol's iodine, 5 drops every 6 h, beginning 4 h after starting propylthiouracil (not before or thyroid hormone stores may be increased). This inhibits further release of thyroxine.

HOMEOSTATIC DECOMPENSATION

• Supportive measures including O_2 and intravenous fluids.
• Treat hyperpyrexia with peripheral cooling measures and paracetemol. Do not use aspirin as it can displace thyroid hormone from its binding sites.
• Give hydrocortisone 100–200 mg i.v. 6-hourly, or dexamethasone 2 mg p.o. 6-hourly.
• Give propranolol 1 mg i.v., repeated every 20 min as necessary up to total of 5 mg; or give 80 mg p.o. four times daily. Be careful if the patient has cardiac failure; rate-dependent failure may improve but patients with a previous history of heart disease may get worse.
• Treat cardiac failure with diuretics.
• Consider digitalization if in atrial fibrillation: note that higher doses of digoxin than usual may be needed due to relative resistance to the drug.

Consider anticoagulation if atrial fibrillation persists, but this is not an immediate priority.

POSSIBLE PRECIPITATING CAUSES

Start broad-spectrum antibiotics if there is any suggestion of infection.

Principles of emergency management of a patient with thyrotoxic crisis:
• Treat the hyperthyroidism.
• Treat homeostatic decompensation including cardiac failure and hyperpyrexia.
• If possible, treat the precipitating event.

See *Endocrinology*, Sections 1.13 and 2.3.
Tietgens ST, Leinung MC. Thyroid storm. *Med Clin North Am* 1995; 79: 169–184.

1.22 Severe headache with meningism

Case history

A 19-year-old male student presents with a day's history of general malaise, anorexia and lethargy. For the last 4 h he has complained of severe headache and neck stiffness.

Clinical approach

Patients with these symptoms range from those who walk into the department to those who are obtunded with cardiorespiratory collapse.
• Assess airway, breathing, circulation.
• If the patient looks unwell, give 100% O$_2$ and obtain venous access.
• Does the patient have meningitis/meningococcal septicaemia or a subarachnoid haemorrhage (SAH)? These are the major concerns and should be your default position.

Consider the differential diagnosis of malaise, headache and neck stiffness (Table 22).

History of the presenting problem

How did the headache start?

Subarachnoid haemorrhage typically presents as a sudden, severe headache unlike any previously experienced.

Are there any other neurological symptoms?

Migraine gives positive symptoms such as auras or visual disturbances that often precede the headache. SAH may give negative symptoms such as visual impairment or weakness that follow the headache. Meningitis is not typically associated with neurological symptoms.

Have there been other symptoms?

Has the patient had a 'flu-like illness with aching muscles and joints? Have they had fevers or sweats? These would be consistent with meningitis, or with 'flu!

Table 22 Differential diagnosis of malaise, headache and neck stiffness.

Common	Must consider
Meningitis	Subarachnoid haemorrhage (Fig. 40)
URTI/'flu	Encephalitis (Fig. 41)
Otitis media	Malaria
Migraine	

URTI, upper respiratory tract infection.

Migraine is almost always associated with nausea and often with vomiting.

Have there been any changes in behaviour or personality? These would be most uncommon, but if present might indicate encephalitis. The patient may be unaware of subtle changes, but these might be noted by friends or family.

Other important points

Ask about the following:
• Any recent problems with the ears or throat?
• Any contact with meningitis?
• Has the patient been abroad recently?
• Is there any personal or family history of migraine, SAH or associated conditions (e.g. adult polycystic kidney disease, heritable connective tissue diseases).

Examination

 Consider meningococcal septicaemia/meningitis.

Look carefully for:
• Rash (Fig. 39)—in the early stages this may be erythematous and macular, only becoming purpuric with time.
• Fundal, subconjunctival or sublingual haemorrhages.
• Nail bed infarcts—a single lesion can make the diagnosis.

Aside from looking for indications of meningococcal disease, the most important aspects are:
• General—temperature; throat and ears for evidence of infection.
• Cardiovascular—pulse rate, blood pressure (lying and sitting) and venous pressure. Is there intravascular volume depletion with postural hypotension? Is the situation

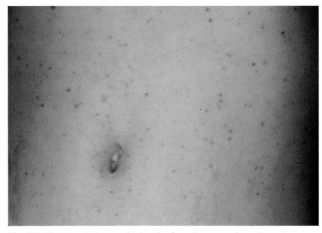

Fig. 39 Characteristic petechial rash of meningococcal septicaemia.

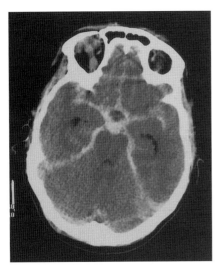

Fig. 40 Unenhanced CT scan of subarachnoid haemorrhage showing blood outlining the circle of Willis.

worse: are there signs of shock with supine hypotension, pallor, clamminess and abnormal capillary refill?

• Neurological—assess for photophobia, neck stiffness and Kernig's test for meningism.

• GCS and brief neurological assessment including fundi, looking for subhyaloid haemorrhages or papilloedema due to raised intracranial pressure.

Approach to investigations and management

 If meningitis is likely, give an appropriate antibiotic immediately.

For most adults in most situations a third-generation cephalosporin would be appropriate, e.g. cefotaxime 2 g i.v. stat, then 4–8-hourly; or ceftriaxone 2 g i.v. stat, then 12-hourly.

Investigations

The following should be checked immediately:

• BM stix—in anyone who is acutely ill or with impaired consciousness.

• Full blood count, electrolytes, glucose, renal and liver function and clotting.

• Blood cultures.

• Cultures taken from scratchings of the skin lesions of meningococcal septicaemia: these often provide the diagnosis, remaining positive after antibiotics have been given.

• Chest radiograph, ECG, arterial blood gases if SAH, meningitis/septicaemia or encephalitis likely.

• Urine dipstick—immune complex deposition in the kidneys can produce dipstick blood and protein.

 SAH can cause neurogenic pulmonary oedema and a variety of ECG changes. The latter may mimic acute coronary ischaemia.

CT scanning

A CT scan never made anyone better—when meningitis is a possible diagnosis it should be performed only after initial management has been instituted, and then only if the patient is stable enough to transfer to the scanner. The patient must be accompanied by suitably trained staff.

Lumbar puncture

In cases of suspected meningitis and encephalitis, lumbar puncture should ideally be performed only after a clear CT scan. In cases of suspected SAH where the CT scan is non-diagnostic, lumbar puncture is indicated.

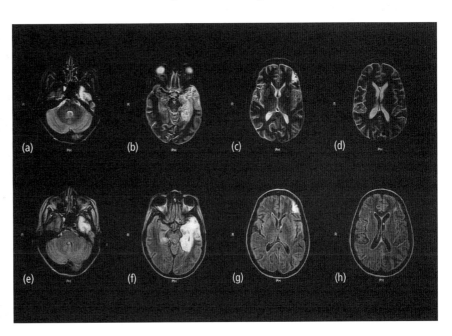

Fig. 41 MRI of herpes simplex encephalitis showing classic cortical distribution in the temporal and parietal lobes with some occipital involvement. (a–d) T2-weighted images; (e–h) fluid-attenuated inverse response (FLAIR) images.

Management

This should comprise supportive care with high-flow O_2 and appropriate fluid resuscitation (see Section 1.11, p. 38), using a urinary catheter to monitor output. Is the patient well, ill, very ill or nearly dead? If the latter—call ICU immediately. Remember that patients with meningococcal disease can 'go off' very rapidly. They need to be kept under continuous observation and an 'isolation room' on a ward is unlikely to be the best place for them.

Antibiotics/antivirals

Give antibiotics and antivirals to too many patients rather than to too few in this context:
• Two suggested regimens are cefotaxime 2 g stat i.v., then 4–8-hourly or ceftriaxone 2 g stat i.v., then 2 g bd, but local microbiological advice may vary.
• Add ampicillin 2 g qds in the very old or immunocompromised to cover *Listeria*.
• Add acyclovir 10 mg/kg tds (adjusted if renal impairment) if herpes simplex encephalitis is a possibility.

See Section 1.2, p. 6; *Infectious diseases*, Sections 1.2, 1.14 and 1.15; *Neurology*, Sections 1.19 and 2.6.
Edlow JA, Caplan LR. Avoiding pitfalls in the diagnosis of subarachnoid haemorrhage. *N Engl J Med* 2000; 349: 29–36.

1.23 Acute spastic paraparesis

Case history

A 38-year-old woman presents with a 3-day history of bilateral leg weakness and tingling.

Clinical approach

Acute onset of lower limb weakness requires urgent diagnosis and management. Time is of the essence if there is a compressive lesion of the spinal cord. The commonest causes are shown in Table 23.

History of the presenting problem

Which of the conditions listed in Table 23 is most likely?

Symptoms of cord compression

Speed and progression of the weakness

Cord compression is usually acute, producing non-progressive and asymmetric weakness. Guillain–Barré syndrome typically presents as weakness, initially distal, that progresses proximally more or less symmetrically over a few days.

Presence or absence of back pain

Sudden onset of pain suggests a herniated disc, spinal subarachnoid haemorrhage or aortic dissection.

Sensory symptoms

Sensory symptoms often precede weakness in cord compression, whereas in Guillain–Barré syndrome they usually come at the same time or afterwards.

Bladder and bowels

Urinary or bowel dysfunction suggests cord compression.

Common	Cord compression	Primary/secondary tumour
		Herniated disc
	Other	Guillain–Barré syndrome
		Transverse myelitis (idiopathic, MS, SLE, PAN, Behçet's, HIV)
Must consider	Vascular causes	Aortic dissection
		Spinal cord SAH
		Thrombosis of anterior spinal artery
	Cord compression	Epidural abscess
		Osteomyelitis (including TB)
	Other	Deficiency diseases (B_{12} deficiency, beriberi, alcoholic neuropathy)
Rare		Toxic polyneuropathies
		Severe hypokalaemia
		Tick paralysis
		Porphyric polyneuropathy

Table 23 Causes of acute or subacute paraplegia/quadriplegia.

HIV, human immunodeficiency virus; MS, multiple sclerosis; PAN, polyarteritis nodosa; SAH, subarachnoid haemorrhage; SLE, systemic lupus erythematosus.

Other symptoms that might give a clue to diagnosis

A thorough history is required:
• Systemic symptoms—anorexia, malaise and weight loss should raise the possibility of underlying malignancy. Fevers, rigors and sweats would point towards osteomyelitis, abscess or TB.
• Systems enquiry—this should be complete, e.g. the comment that 'I've been a bit constipated for the last few months' might mean colonic malignancy.
• Note breathlessness in particular—this is a sinister symptom in Guillain–Barré syndrome that may indicate the need for respiratory support; ventilatory failure can progress very rapidly in this syndrome.

Other relevant past medical history

The important issues are:
• Previous history of malignancy.
• Previous neurological problems, perhaps suggestive of demyelination: have you ever had anything like this before? Have you ever had trouble with your vision?
• Exposure to drugs or toxins.

Examination

General

Examine carefully:
• For evidence of primary malignancy (especially breast) or infection.
• For cardiovascular signs of autonomic dysfunction, which is often a feature of Guillain–Barré syndrome.
• Respiratory function—particularly important for patients with suspected Guillain–Barré syndrome. 'Take a deep breath and count out loud as far as you can … 1, 2, 3, 4 and so on'. How far the patient can count correlates fairly well with their forced vital capacity: and the test can easily be repeated to see if they are getting better or worse.
• Can you feel the bladder?

Neurological

Look for features of cord compression:
• Is there a sensory level? Below the level of a lesion there will be sensory loss: be obsessional about trying to find this. Incomplete lesions, where there is not a sharp cut-off between normal and paralysis/sensory deficit, have a much better prognosis.
• Below the level of the lesion there will be weakness, increased tone and hyperreflexia. Do the plantars go up or down?

• Weakness that is most marked at the ankles with sensory loss in the saddle area and sphincter disturbance suggests a cauda equina lesion.
• The presence of neurological signs above the level of a cord lesion, e.g. optic atrophy, suggests demyelination or a systemic aetiology (see Table 23).

The patient with urinary retention:
 Patients with cord compression can present with acute urinary retention but little objective leg weakness. A common error is to omit assessment of the sacral dermatomes in someone with urinary retention: 'shove a catheter in—it must be the prostate'. When performing the rectal examination in someone with retention, always ask 'can you feel me touching you here?' before you start.

Approach to investigations and immediate management

Investigations

The following investigations should be requested urgently:
• FBC, U & Es, LFTs, Ca^{2+}/PO_4^{2-}, glucose, ESR, immunoglobulins and clotting screen.
• Urine for Bence-Jones protein.
• Radiograph of spine at the appropriate level.
• Chest radiograph.
• Respiratory function tests and arterial blood gases if Guillain–Barré syndrome is suspected.

Imaging and lumbar puncture

MRI is the study of choice for non-traumatic paraplegia or quadriplegia (Fig. 42) and should be requested as an emergency.

A CT scan and/or a myelogram may be indicated in individual patients, but CT scanning alone may not exclude cord compression and myelography carries the risk of clinical deterioration in cases of cord compression.

Lumbar puncture should not be performed until spinal cord compression has been eliminated as a possibility.

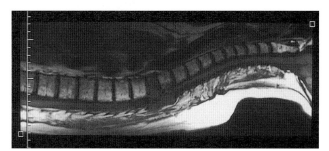
Fig. 42 MRI study, T2-weighted image, showing a spinal secondary deposit with compression of the cord.

Initial treatment

Your immediate priorities are to:
• Relieve urinary retention.
• Place the patient on a pressure-relieving mattress.
• Monitor pulse oximetry, respiratory function (peak flow rate or FEV$_1$) and ECG if Guillain–Barré syndrome is a possibility.
• Involve the specialists early—expeditious surgery can prevent permanent paralysis and high-dose steroids have been shown to be of benefit if given within 8 h of acute spinal cord injury.

• The diagnosis of cord compression must not be missed.
• Speed of diagnosis and treatment is vital if permanent paraplegia is to be avoided.
• Early specialist referral is fundamental in management.

See *Neurology*, Sections 1.11, 1.13 and 2.5.
Bracken MB, Shepard MJ, Collins WF. A randomised, controlled trial of methylprednisolone or naloxone in the treatment of acute spinal cord injury. *N Engl J Med* 1990; 322: 1405–1411.
Kurtztke JF. Epidemiology of spinal cord injury. *Exp Neurol* 1975; 48: 163–236.
Swain A, Grundy D, Russell J. *ABC of Spinal Cord Injury*. London: BMJ Publications, 1986.

1.24 Status epilepticus

Case history

A 50-year-old man has been found collapsed and fitting in the street. By the time he arrives in hospital he has been fitting continuously for 40 minutes.

Clinical approach

Immediately:
• Assess airway, breathing, circulation.
• Check the BM stix.
• Give 100% O$_2$.
• Secure intravenous access.

The prognosis of status epilepticus is related to its duration. Priority should then be given to terminating the fit:
• If the BM is low, give 50 mL 50% dextrose i.v.
• Give 10 mg diazepam i.v., repeated after 5 min if no response. If intravenous access cannot be obtained, diazepam can be given rectally.

Table 24 Causes of status epilepticus. Pseudofits should only be considered when organic pathology is definitely excluded.

Common	Must consider
Primary epilepsy	Space-occupying lesion
Hypoglycaemia	Anoxia
SAH/CVA	Intracerebral infection and meningitis
Alcohol/drug withdrawal	Other metabolic disturbance, e.g. hyponatraemia, uraemia

SAH, subarachnoid haemorrhage; CVA, cerebrovascular accident.

• If no response after 20 mg diazepam, give 15 mg/kg phenytoin i.v. (at a rate of no more than 50 mg/min). If the patient is known to be on phenytoin, try phenobarbitone 15 mg/kg (at a rate of no more than 100 mg/min).
• If no response, call an anaesthetist—the patient may need to be fully anaesthetized.
• Consider possible underlying causes for status epilepticus (Table 24).

Inserting an oral airway during a fit is almost impossible and likely to damage teeth or soft tissue. It is better to wait until the fit subsides.

History of the presenting problem

The patient cannot talk, but:
• Have they got a Medic Alert bracelet or necklace?
• Have they got anything in their pockets that suggests they are an epileptic (or diabetic), e.g. medication, outpatient attendance cards, etc.

Get as much history as possible from the ambulance crew and accompanying persons.
• Is the patient a known epileptic?
• What is their regular medication? Do they have any allergies?
• If they do take anticonvulsants, have there been any recent changes in medication that may have altered the levels? Or intercurrent illness that may have prevented the patient taking or absorbing their tablets, e.g. vomiting?
• Is there other significant past medical history?
• Is there any evidence of alcohol or drug abuse or overdose?

Examination

Examine thoroughly for evidence of precipitating pathology and for signs of alcohol or drug abuse. Also check the mouth and tongue: there can be horrible damage and swelling after a fit and anaesthetic help may be needed in order to secure the airway.

Your comprehensive neurological examination will include a record of:

- GCS
- pupil size and reaction
- other brain-stem signs (see Section 1.26, p. 75)
- symmetry of tone and reflexes in the limbs
- focal neurological abnormalities that may suggest localized pathology—but remember Todd's paresis which can cause confusion.

Approach to investigations and management

Investigations

These should include:
- Urgent FBC, U & Es and glucose; save a sample for measurement of anticonvulsant levels.
- Creatine phosphokinase—if there has been prolonged fitting and there is a risk of rhabdomyolysis.
- Sepsis screen—chest radiograph; urine dipstick and M,C & S.
- ECG.
- Arterial blood gases.
- Toxicology screen, CT scan and lumbar puncture for selected patients.

Treatment

This follows your immediate management aimed at terminating the fit:
- Nurse in the recovery position, with an oropharyngeal airway and near to suction in case of vomiting.
- Continue to give high-flow O_2, and monitor with pulse oximetry and ECG.
- Intravenous fluids.
- Urinary catheterization.
- Broad-spectrum antibiotics and/or antivirals if there is any possibility of infection.
- Half-hourly neuro-observations.
- A pressure-relieving mattress.

> The patient who does not wake up:
> - In prolonged uncontrolled epilepsy the fits can become progressively more subtle, perhaps just abnormal eye movements in someone remaining unconconscious. This is called non-convulsive status epilepticus and may go unnoticed.
> - Consider an EEG in any seriously ill patient with coma of unclear cause.

See Sections 1.17 (p. 57) and 1.26 (p. 75); *Gastroenterology*, Section 1; *Neurology*, Sections 1.7 and 2.12.
Cochius J. Status epilepticus. *CPD J Intern Med* 1999; (1): 3–8.
Delanty N, Vaughan CJ, French JA. Medical causes of seizures. *Lancet* 1998; 352: 383–390.

1.25 Stroke

Case history

An 80-year-old woman presents with sudden onset of weakness of her right side and slurred speech. Her husband, who had been in the kitchen, returned to the living room to find her slumped in an armchair.

Clinical approach

Acute stroke is one of the commonest medical emergencies. Secondary brain injury often results from failure to attend comprehensively to the resuscitation of these patients. Your priorities are:
- Assess airway, breathing, circulation.
- Check a blood sugar and treat hypoglycaemia promptly.
- Check GCS: patients with a GCS <12 may benefit from a nasal or oral airway; those with a GCS <8 need to be considered for elective intubation.
- Give high-flow O_2 and obtain intravenous access.
- Rapid assessment of the neurological disability: is her slurred speech in fact dysphasia?
- Consider the differential diagnosis of stroke (Table 25). Is the patient pyrexial? If so, consider unusual cerebral pathology such as brain abscess or meningitis and secondary causes of fever, particularly aspiration or hypostatic pneumonia.

History of the presenting problem

After rapid initial assessment, continue as described below.

Can the patient give you a history? It may be that she is dysphasic. If what she is saying and the way she responds to you seem in any way unusual, then test formally for this immediately:
- 'I am having difficulty understanding what you are saying.'

Table 25 Differential diagnosis of stroke.

Common	Must consider
Thrombotic stroke	Subdural haematoma
Embolic stroke	Giant cell arteritis
Subarachnoid haemorrhage	Hypoglycaemia
	Aortic/carotid dissection
	Encephalitis/meningitis
	Cerebral abscess
	Cerebral tumour (primary or secondary)

• 'Would it be alright for me to check one or two things?'
• 'Can you tell me your name and address?' Someone with significant dysphasia is unlikely to be able to do this in an entirely normal way.
• 'Can you open your mouth … show me your hand … touch your nose?' Give tasks of increasing complexity to find out if there is receptive dysphasia.

If she (or her husband) can give a history, then enquire regarding:
• Preceding symptoms. Consider again the differential diagnosis of stroke in Table 25. Are there any clues? A sudden, severe headache suggests subarachnoid haemorrhage. Jaw pain and temporal tenderness suggests giant cell arteritis. Weakness of gradual onset would suggest a space-occupying lesion.
• Have you ever had anything like this before? Ask particularly about amaurosis fugax and transient ischaemic attacks: have you ever had trouble with the vision in one of your eyes? Have you ever had weakness in the arm or leg that lasted for a short while only?
• Is there any known previous medical history, especially of cardiovascular disease, peripheral vascular disease, diabetes or hypertension?
• What is the patient's normal level of functioning? Do they need assistance with activities of daily living? What are the social circumstances?
• Drugs and allergies.
• Smoking history.

Examination

General

Thorough general examination is required, checking in particular for the following:
• Pyrexia.
• Neck stiffness—likely to indicate blood in the CSF; either due to primary subarachnoid haemorrhage or (more likely) secondary to intracerebral bleeding.
• Cardiovascular—heart rate and rhythm: is she in atrial fibrillation? Are there any murmurs? Measure blood pressure, but remember that 'hypertension' is difficult to define just after a stroke. Is there evidence of peripheral vascular disease, i.e. absent peripheral pulses and arterial bruits?
• Respiratory—adequacy of ventilation and evidence of aspiration.

Neurological

The important issues are to:
• Check GCS.
• Determine the approximate site of the lesion, and the degree of neurological deficit. In particular, document the

presence or absence of a gag reflex—should the patient be allowed to eat and drink?

Although patients with a GCS of <8 are at high risk of aspiration, a proportion of patients with higher GCS will have lost their gag reflex.
The ability to swallow should be checked formally by administration of thickened fluids, and patients with stroke should be put 'nil by mouth' until this has been done.

Approach to investigations and management

Investigations

The following are required urgently:
• FBC, U & Es, glucose, CRP or ESR.
• Chest radiograph.
• ECG—exclude dysrhythmias and look for evidence of acute myocardial infarction.
• CT scan of brain—is this haemorrhage or a space-occupying lesion? With an infarct the appearances are likely to be subtle, and the scan might be entirely normal.

Stroke can be the presenting feature of approximately 5% of myocardial infarctions in the elderly.

Emergency management

Do all that you can to prevent secondary brain damage.

Oxygen

Normalize arterial O_2 saturation, which may be impaired due to aspiration, atelectasis or a reduced central drive to ventilation.

Intravenous fluids

These should be administered unless a gag reflex is present and the patient is able to request and take oral fluids.

Blood pressure

Blood pressure commonly increases following acute stroke and settles over the next 24–48 h. Immediate treatment is not usually appropriate: cerebral autoregulation is disturbed and aggressive attempts to reduce the blood pressure are more likely to do harm than good. However, if the systolic is consistently above 220 mmHg or the diastolic above 130 mmHg, most physicians with an interest in stroke would recommend gentle pressure reduction. Modified release nifedipine 10 mg p.o. stat would be a suitable initial treatment.

In stroke associated with malignant hypertension, the blood pressure needs to be lowered slowly over a period of hours.

Glycaemic control

Control of hyperglycaemia should be achieved with intravenous insulin using a sliding scale. Good glycaemic control improves the outcome from acute stroke.

Aspirin

Aspirin should be given when haemorrhagic stroke has been excluded.

Other important aspects of management

Nurse the patient on a pressure-relieving mattress. A urinary catheter may be required. Refer the patient early to ancillary services—speech therapy, physiotherapy, occupational therapy and the social work department.

It is vital to assess and clearly record the patient's resuscitation status: this decision should be made by a senior member of the medical team. Information about the patient's quality of life before the stroke will clearly be relevant.

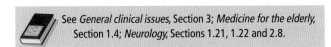
See *General clinical issues*, Section 3; *Medicine for the elderly*, Section 1.4; *Neurology*, Sections 1.21, 1.22 and 2.8.

1.26 Coma

Case history

A 40-year-old man has been found collapsed in his flat where he lives alone. He has not been seen for 2 days. He is unconscious.

Clinical approach

Prioritize as follows:
• Assess airway, breathing, circulation.
• Give 100% O_2, monitor pulse oximetry and obtain venous access.
• Record the GCS and check the pupil size and reaction.
• Check the BM and the temperature.
• Consider the differential diagnosis (Table 26).
• Look for a Medic Alert bracelet or necklace.

Table 26 Differential diagnosis of collapse and coma.

Common	Must consider
Poisoning; alcohol, opiates, tricyclics, benzodiazepines. Also carbon monoxide (accidental or deliberate)	Sepsis (systemic or intracerebral) Severe metabolic disturbance Status epilepticus (non-convulsive)
Hypoglycaemia	
SAH	
CVA	
Head injury	
Postictal	
Hypothermia	

CVA, cerebrovascular accident; SAH, subarachnoid haemorrhage.

 Glasgow Coma Scale

Best eye opening response	Score
Spontaneously	4
To speech	3
To pain	2
None	1
Best verbal response	
Orientated	5
Confused conversation	4
Words	3
Sounds	2
None	1
Best motor response	
Obeys commands	6
Localization to painful stimuli	5
Withdraws to pain	4
Flexor (decorticate) response to pain	3
Extensor (decerebrate) response to pain	2
No response	1

Notes. Painful stimuli: rub knuckles on sternum, apply pressure to nail bed, e.g. by squeezing pencil or biro against it. Do not use methods that might lead to bleeding or bruising, e.g. pins, supraorbital pressure.

Motor response should be scored as the best response of any limb.

Overall response is graded by adding the scores in the three areas: maximum (normal) = 15; minimum = 3; coma is defined as 8 or less; significant deterioration is defined as a decrease in GCS score of 2 or more.

Immediate therapy includes:
• If BM is low, give 50 mL 50% dextrose i.v.
• If pupils are small, respiratory rate is low or signs of drug abuse are present, give 400 µg naloxone i.v. stat, repeating the dose as necessary to a total of 1.2 mg if there is any suggestion of response.
• If hypothermic, start rewarming.

 The half lives of most opiates are longer than that of naloxone, therefore repeated doses or an infusion may be required.

Any patient with prolonged immobility may develop:
- rhabdomyolysis
- pressure necrosis
- compartment syndromes
- secondary hypothermia/sepsis.

History of the presenting problem

From the ambulance crew or accompanying persons, discover:
- The circumstances in which the patient was found. Was there anything to suggest carbon monoxide poisoning? Were drug bottles or syringes nearby? Was there a suicide note?
- When was the person last seen?
- Is there a known past medical history, medication or allergies?
- Possible alcohol or drug use.

The most important pieces of equipment in such cases are a six-inch nail and a hammer. The nail should be driven through the shoes of the ambulance crew to prevent them from leaving until a full history has been obtained.
(Anon)

Examination

After immediate check of airway, breathing, circulation and GCS and treatment of hypoglycaemia and opiate overdose, a thorough assessment of all systems is essential. Concentrate on the following.

Respiratory rate and pattern

This is an important clue to aetiology and is often overlooked. Consider the following.
- Cheyne–Stokes respiration is commonly associated with bilateral cortical damage.
- Hyperventilation may occur secondary to metabolic acidosis (see Section 1.19, p. 62), pulmonary pathology or rarely with brain-stem pathology.
- Bizarre respiratory patterns may be associated with brain-stem pathology [1].

Pupil size and reaction

The brain-stem areas controlling consciousness are anatomically adjacent to those controlling the pupils—and pupillary changes are a valuable guide to the presence and location of brain-stem pathology resulting in coma:
- Bilateral, fixed and dilated pupils suggest severe damage and are a poor prognostic sign.
- A unilateral, fixed and dilated pupil indicates a third nerve lesion, commonly due to uncal herniation from a

supratentorial mass lesion or a posterior communicating artery aneurysm.
- Unilateral Horner's syndrome suggests damage to the hypothalamus or a lateral medullary/syndrome.
- Bilateral, small pupils suggest pontine damage or opiate overdose.

Spontaneous eye movements

- Abnormal conjugate deviation suggests intracerebral damage.
- Dysconjugate deviation implies damage to nerves III, IV or VI.

Always consider Wernicke's syndrome (see Section 1.14, p. 47) and if there is any possibility of this, give 100 mg thiamine i.v. and check serum magnesium (a cofactor for the enzyme).

Peripheral tone and reflexes

Asymmetry suggests focal neurological damage.

Approach to investigations and management

Investigations

Immediately organize:
- FBC, U & Es, glucose, renal and liver function tests.
- Chest radiograph (aspiration?).
- ECG—beware 'ischaemic' changes in subarachnoid haemorrhage.
- Sepsis screen (blood cultures; urine dipstick and M,C & S).
- Arterial blood gases (see Section 1.19, p. 62).
- A CT or MRI scan of the brain will be required as an urgent investigation in any patient who is comatose for unknown reason. This may reveal something that requires immediate neurosurgical attention, e.g. some extradural, subdural or intracerebral haematomas, and all cases with these conditions should be discussed with a neurosurgeon.
- A lumbar puncture will be required, after CT scan, in selected patients.

Management

The following emergency measures are general requirements of the comatose patient:
- Protected airway.
- High-flow O_2.
- Intravenous fluids.
- Urinary catheter.

- Broad-spectrum antibiotics and/or antivirals should be given empirically if there is any suggestion of bacterial infection or encephalitis (see Section 1.22, p. 68).
- Half-hourly neuro-observations.
- A suitable pressure-relieving mattress.

The patient's resuscitation status must be considered and recorded when a specific diagnosis has been established and prognosis assessed.

Treatment of specific causes of coma will be required and these are discussed in other sections of this module:
Overdoses. See Section 2.1, p. 83.
Stroke. See Section 1.25, p. 73.
Hypoglycaemia. See Section 1.17, p. 57.
Meningitis and Encephalitis. See Section 1.22, p. 68.
Hypothermia. See Section 1.6, p. 22.
Subarachnoid haemorrhage. See Section 1.22, p. 68.
Status epilepticus. See Section 1.24, p. 72.

1 Plum F, Posner JB. *The Diagnosis of Stupor and Coma*, 3rd edn. Philadelphia: F.A. Davis Co., 1980.
2 Jenkins PF. Coma. *CPD Journal of Internal Medicine* 1999; 1(2). Rila Publications Ltd, pp. 43–49.

1.27 Fever in a returning traveller

Case history

A 25-year-old man is brought to A&E by his friends. He has recently returned from a back-packing trip around Thailand and has not been well since his return. He is drowsy and has a temperature of 39°C.

Clinical approach

If any patient is drowsy and unwell, organize management as follows:
- Check airway, breathing, circulation.
- Check GCS.
- Administer high-flow O_2 and monitor pulse oximetry.
- Monitor heart rate and rhythm.
- Establish intravenous access.
- Check the BM stix estimation of glucose.

And in this case consider the differential diagnosis of fever and coma in a returning traveller (Table 27).

Malaria:
- Consider malaria in any patient presenting to hospital with a relevant travel history.
- There are no diagnostic findings on examination.
- Missing the diagnosis can be fatal.

Table 27 Causes of fever and coma in the returning traveller.

Malaria	—
Other infections causing fever and coma	Viral, bacterial, fungal, protozoal (other than malaria) or helminthic meningoencephalitis Cerebral abscess
Any cause of fever with any cause of coma	e.g. 'flu with hypoglycaemia e.g. pneumonia with opiate overdose

See *Infectious diseases*, Sections 1.20, 1.22 and 1.23.

History of the presenting problem

A full history is required, but a detailed travel history is obviously of particular importance. What pathogens might the patient may have been exposed to? Enquire from the patient and/or his companions regarding:
- countries visited, with dates
- areas visited—were they rural or urban, rainforest or savannah?
- accommodation used
- activities whilst there, e.g. freshwater exposure, trekking
- exposure to animals
- sexual history
- vaccinations received prior to travel
- antimalarial chemoprophylaxis and compliance.

Examination

How ill is the patient? Well, ill, very ill or nearly dead? If the latter, get ICU help immediately.

Cardiovascular system

Check peripheral perfusion, pulse, blood pressure (lying and sitting), JVP, heart sounds, lung bases and peripheral oedema. If shocked, start resuscitation immediately whilst completing the history and examination.

Other

Examine other systems, in this case looking specifically for the following:
- rash
- anaemia
- jaundice
- bleeding
- lymphadenopathy
- hepatosplenomegaly.

Coma and fever from abroad— differential diagnosis

Malaria

Cerebral malaria, which is a complication of *Plasmodium*

falciparum infection, may present with coma. Malaria must be the working diagnosis in all patients with possible exposure who present with coma and/or fever until proved otherwise. There will probably be an antecedent history of a short, febrile illness with rigors and headache. Anaemia and slight jaundice are common, with moderate tender hepatosplenomegaly. There is no rash or lymphadenopathy. Urgent treatment is essential, therefore blood films for malaria parasites should be performed immediately in any patient with these symptoms who has visited a malarious area within the last 6 months.

Other diagnoses

The diagnosis is malaria! But consider other diagnoses listed in Table 27 and discussed in more detail in *Infectious diseases*, Sections 1.20, 1.22 and 1.23.

Approach to investigations and management

- Do not tackle this on your own!
- If malaria, get advice from an appropriate specialist in infectious diseases regarding management.
- If not malaria and not obviously falling into the group headed 'any cause of fever with any cause of coma' in Table 27, get help from an appropriate specialist in infectious disease to try to make a diagnosis.

Investigations

- All patients should have an immediate malaria film (Fig. 43) even if they have taken chemoprophylaxis (see *Infectious diseases*, Sections 2.13.1 and 3.1). Remember that a single negative film does not exclude malaria.
- Check full blood count, glucose, electrolytes, renal and liver function tests and coagulation screen—anaemia, leucopenia, thrombocytopenia, renal failure, deranged liver function and abnormal clotting may all be seen with malaria.

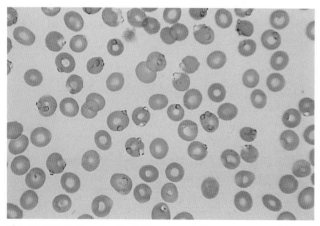

Fig. 43 Malaria film showing falciparum malaria.

- Always take blood cultures from a patient with undiagnosed fever.
- Chest radiograph—look for signs of infection (perhaps due to aspiration in someone who is drowsy) or pulmonary oedema, a complication of malaria.
- Other tests will be required to make a diagnosis if that of malaria cannot be sustained (see Sections 1.22, p. 68, 1.26, p. 75 and *Infectious diseases*, Section 1.20).

Emergency management of malaria

Falciparum malaria is usually the cause of severe, complicated malaria. Patients infected with *P. vivax*, *P. ovale* or *P. malariae* tend to have milder symptoms. Remember that vivax and ovale malaria can cause symptoms for the first time more than 12 months after infection.

The emergency management of severe malaria is described below.

Supportive measures

Patients with malaria may be seriously ill and require admission to the ICU.
- Give O$_2$ and monitor pulse oximetry.
- Is intravascular volume depleted? If there is hypotension or postural hypotension with low venous pressure, then resuscitate immediately (see Section 1.11, p. 38). Monitor fluid balance carefully. Put in a central line (after volume expansion) and urinary catheter.
- Hypoglycaemia is common in severe malaria—monitor blood glucose hourly and give intravenous dextrose if necessary.
- Remember that bacterial infection may coexist with malaria—if the patient is seriously ill, treat empirically with a broad-spectrum antibiotic after taking blood cultures.

Drug treatment

FALCIPARUM MALARIA

- Quinine dihydrochloride is the drug of choice.
- Give a loading dose of 20 mg/kg (maximum 1.4 g) in 5% dextrose i.v. over 4 h, followed by maintenance therapy of 10 mg/kg (maximum 700 mg) in 5% dextrose over 4 h tds.
- Omit the loading dose if the patient is on mefloquine or quinine has been given in the last 24 h.
- Make sure that the patient is on a cardiac monitor and the blood glucose is measured hourly while quinine is being administered.
- Seek expert advice as soon as possible if the patient has been to northern Thailand, Laos or Burma as there is a high incidence of quinine resistance in these areas and combination therapy may be required.

- If the patient has mild symptoms and can tolerate oral therapy prescribe oral quinine dihydrochloride sulphate 600 mg 8-hourly.
- After 7 days of treatment with quinine give a single dose of 3 tablets of Fansidar (sulfadoxine/pyramethamine), or doxycycline 100 mg daily for 7 days.

VIVAX, OVALE AND MALARIAE MALARIA

Give oral chloroquine 600 mg immediately, followed after 6 h by 300 mg, then two further doses of 300 mg at 24-h intervals.

In vivax and ovale infections chloroquine should then be followed by a 2-week course of primaquine, 15 mg daily, to eliminate parasites from the liver.

 Remember to screen patients for glucose-6-phosphate dehydrogenase deficiency before giving primaquine otherwise severe haemolysis may ensue.

Treatment of complications

CEREBRAL MALARIA

Organize a CT head scan followed by a lumbar puncture (if not contraindicated): it is important to exclude other infectious causes of coma. Consider prophylactic phenobarbitone to prevent seizures.

RENAL FAILURE

Renal replacement therapy may be required.

SEVERE ANAEMIA

Anaemia is common and rarely requires treatment, but if severe and associated with a heavy parasite load (>10%), exchange transfusion may be indicated.

DISSEMINATED INTRAVASCULAR COAGULATION

This should be treated in the usual way (see *Haematology*, Section 2.4).

 See *Infectious diseases*, Sections 1.20, 2.13.1 and 3.1. Felton JM, Bryceson ADM. Fever in the returning traveller. *Br J Hosp Med* 1996; 55: 705–711. Svenson JE, MacLean JD, Gyorkos TW, Keystone J. Imported malaria. *Arch Intern Med* 1995; 155: 861–867.

1.28 Septicaemia

Case history

A 75-year-old woman is brought to A&E after she has been found wandering in the street in her nightclothes. Her daughter tells you that she is normally mentally alert and enjoys completing the *Guardian* crossword every day. She is drowsy and confused with a temperature of 39°C.

Clinical approach

Acute confusional state, with or without pyrexia, in a previously well elderly person indicates sepsis until proved otherwise. Urgent treatment is essential if the patient is very ill:
- Check airway, breathing, circulation and GCS.
- Give high-flow O_2 and monitor oximetry and ECG.
- Check the blood sugar by BM stix, ratified by subsequent laboratory blood sugar estimation.
- Establish intravenous access. If the patient is shocked start intravenous fluids immediately.
- Consider the differential diagnosis of confusion in the elderly (Table 28).
- Take blood cultures, then start empirical treatment with intravenous antibiotics immediately even if there is no obvious source of infection.

History of the presenting problem

In this context, the patient will usually be unable to give a coherent history. Try to gain as much information as possible from relatives and friends in an attempt to determine the source of infection (Table 29). Ask specifically regarding the following:
- History of cough, dysuria, abdominal pain and leg ulcers.
- Recent history of surgery or trauma.
- Relevant past medical history that may enhance susceptibility to infection, e.g. diabetes, chronic obstructive pulmonary disease, valvular heart disease, venous ulcers or an indwelling urinary catheter.

Table 28 Causes of confusion in the elderly. Note that any cause of serious illness can lead to confusion.

Infection
Drugs, e.g. benzodiazepines, tricyclic antidepressants, anticholinergics
Constipation/urinary retention
Hypoglycaemia
Alcohol withdrawal
Organ failure, e.g. cardiorespiratory (hypoxia), renal failure, liver failure
Electrolyte disturbance, e.g. hyponatraemia, hypercalcaemia
Cerebrovascular disease, e.g. stroke

Table 29 Possible sources of infection in a patient with sepsis.

Common	Less common
Pneumonia	Loculated pus—abscess anywhere
Urinary tract	Intra-abdominal—e.g. peritonitis, cholecystitis
Skin—e.g. cellulitis, infected ulcers	Meningitis—never to be forgotten

Note that the list is not exhaustive: there are many other infections! A history of foreign travel immediately brings a much wider differential diagnosis. All have malaria until proved otherwise (see Section 1.27, p. 77). Do not forget iatrogenic sources of infection: urinary catheters, intravenous cannulae, etc.

- Travel history—elderly people do go on exotic holidays.

Examination

Immediate priorities

- What is the general state of the patient? Are they well, ill, very ill or nearly dead? If nearly dead call for ICU help immediately.
- Are they shocked? Check peripheral perfusion, pulse, blood pressure (lying and sitting) and JVP. If they are shocked start resuscitation immediately whilst completing the history and examination (see Section 1.11, p. 38).
- Check other vital signs—temperature and respiratory rate.

Further examination

A thorough examination is required.

General

Look specifically for rash or skin infection.

Cardiovascular

You have already assessed vital signs; now listen for murmurs and look for peripheral stigmata of infectious endocarditis (see *Cardiology*, Section 1.13).

Respiratory

Is there evidence of consolidation or pleural fluid, which might be due to empyema? Note the O_2 saturation, but remember that sepsis can cause hypoxia through the adult respiratory distress syndrome, not just because of a respiratory source of infection.

Abdominal

Look for peritonism, an abdominal mass or an enlarged/ tender abdominal organ, e.g. pyonephrosis or an empyema of the gall bladder. Do not forget the rectal examination; if you do not look you will not find the perianal abscess.

Neurological

You have already assessed conscious level; now check for neck stiffness and photophobia.

Fever in diabetics

Remember to look carefully at the perineum and feet: these are common sites of infection in diabetics.

Consider the following in patients with fever but no obvious source of sepsis:
- Are they neutropenic?
- Are they immunocompromised?
- Are they an intravenous drug user?
- Peritonitis in the elderly can present with fairly unimpressive abdominal signs.

Approach to investigations and management

Investigations

Routine

All patients who might be septic require:
- Full blood count, glucose, electrolytes, renal and liver function and coagulation screen.
- Arterial blood gases—if O_2 saturation <95% on pulse oximetry or the patient is very ill.
- Cultures—blood, urine (dipstick and send sample for microscopy and culture).
- Chest radiograph—look for signs of consolidation or pleural effusion. Remember that a small pleural effusion may be a 'sympathetic' phenomenon and indicate primary pathology under the diaphragm, e.g. a subphrenic abscess or an empyema of the gall bladder.

The normal white cell count

The white cell count is normal in patients who are well, but can also be normal or low in overwhelming bacterial sepsis when it is a sign of poor prognosis.

Remember that a normal white count does not exclude infection.

Other investigations

The clinical picture may demand other investigations: wound swabs, lumbar puncture, joint aspiration, sputum culture, abdominal or pelvic ultrasound.

Table 30 Initial antibiotic choice for severe infections. NB Local antibiotic policies will vary. Consult your hospital policy.

Suspected focus of infection	Initial antibiotic therapy
Severe community-acquired pneumonia	Ceftriaxone 3 g + clarithromycin 500 mg i.v.
Hospital-acquired pneumonia	Ceftriaxone 2 g i.v.
Aspiration pneumonia	Add metronidazole 1 g rectally to above
Complicated UTI/pyelonephritis	Ciprofloxacin 500 mg orally or gentamicin 5 mg/kg if intravenous therapy is necessary
Meningitis	Ceftriaxone 4 g i.v. (+ ampicillin 3 g i.v. if *Listeria* is suspected, e.g. pregnant, elderly, immunocompromised
Severe soft tissue infection	Benzylpenicillin 1.2 g + flucloxacillin 1 g i.v. (clarithromycin 500 mg i.v. if penicillin allergy)
Bone/joint infection	Benzylpenicillin 1.2 g + flucloxacillin 2 g + gentamicin 5 mg/kg i.v.
Peritonitis/intra-abdominal sepsis	Amoxycillin 1 g + gentamicin 5 mg/kg i.v. + metronidazole 1 g rectally (vancomycin instead of amoxycillin if penicillin allergy)
Postoperative wound infection	Cefuroxime 750 mg i.v. + metronidazole 1 g rectally
Life-threatening infection with no source identified	Gentamicin 5 mg/kg + flucloxacillin 2 g + benzylpenicillin 1.2 g i.v. (if hospital-acquired use tazocin 4.5 g)

UTI, urinary tract infection.

Always check for meningism and examine the joints obsessionally. Reduced conscious level in the septic patient should cause you to think hard about the need for head CT scan followed by lumbar puncture.

Management

Resuscitation and supportive measures

This should have been started immediately while taking the history and examining the patient:
• Maintain the airway and give high-flow O_2 via a reservoir mask, using pulse oximetry to monitor PaO_2—if the patient remains hypoxic despite face-mask O_2, intubation and ventilation may be required.
• Establish intravenous access and correct intravascular volume depletion rapidly (see Section 1.11, p. 38). Put in a central line (after initial resuscitation) and urinary catheter to monitor fluid balance. If hypotension persists despite an adequate CVP, consider inotropic support, e.g. norepinephrine (noradrenaline), dopamine or enoximone after discussion with colleagues from the ICU ('would you like to take this patient now … or later?').
• Anticipate that prerenal renal failure or acute tubular necrosis is likely. If the CVP has risen into the range 5–8 cm, do not continue to give large volumes of fluid if the urine output is low: you will induce fluid overload and pulmonary oedema. Give daily fluid input equal to the last 24 h output plus allowance (0.5–1 L) for insensible losses. Check fluid status clinically at least twice daily and adjust fluid regimen accordingly. Consider indications for renal replacement therapy (see Section 1.15, p. 52 and *Nephrology*, Sections 1.6 and 1.7).
• Anticipate disseminated intravascular coagulation (DIC). Seek advice from a haematologist if there is active bleeding.

Is DIC present? Does the patient need fresh frozen plasma and/or platelets?
• Continue to monitor blood sugar with BM stix—a low blood sugar is common in sepsis.

Antibiotic therapy

Empirical broad-spectrum antibiotics are the order of the day. Do not wait to confirm sepsis before starting them. The specific choice of antibiotics will be dictated by the clinical picture (Table 30).

Removal of infective focus

The following are basic—but still sometimes forgotten, so no apologies for mentioning them:
• remove any urinary catheter, intravenous cannula or central line that may be a source of infection
• get a surgical opinion if an abdominal or pelvic collection is suspected
• refer for incision and drainage of any superficial abscess, or debridement of infected tissue.

Principles of emergency management in a patient with sepsis are:
• resuscitation and supportive measures
• antibiotic therapy
• removal of infective focus.

See Section 1.27, p. 77; *Infectious Diseases*, Sections 1.1, 1.2 and 1.15.

1.29 Anaphylaxis

Case history

A 40-year-old woman complains of difficulty breathing and has swollen lips and tongue. The symptoms started a few minutes after she took a tablet of amoxycillin for an infected wisdom tooth.

Clinical approach

- Assess airway, breathing, circulation.
- The clinical history suggests anaphylaxis, with the risk of rapidly developing life-threatening airway obstruction, bronchoconstriction or cardiovascular collapse.
- Get help: more than one pair of hands is necessary. Call for immediate anaesthetic/ICU assistance and summon the cardiac arrest team before rather than after arrest.

Immediate therapy includes:
- 100% O_2.
- Epinephrine (adrenaline), if there is stridor, wheeze, respiratory distress or clinical signs of shock. The initial dose is 0.5 mL 1 : 1000 solution i.m. Repeat in 5 min if there is no clinical improvement.
- Chlorpheniramine 10–20 mg i.m. or i.v.
- Nebulized salbutamol (5–10 mg) if bronchospasm is present.

 For life-threatening anaphylaxis, consider slow, intravenous epinephrine (adrenaline) 1 : 10 000 solution (note the 10-fold dilution compared with the i.m. injection): give 5 ml (0.5 mg) at a rate of 1 ml/min (0.1 mg/min), stopping when a response has been obtained.

History of the presenting problem

If someone presents with anaphylaxis out of the blue, ask:
- Is there a history of allergy to anything?
- Exactly what has been taken and when? Almost anything could be relevant, e.g. minute trace of nut in a restaurant meal specifically stated not to contain nuts.

- Previous medical history, including a drug history.
- Relevant family history—consider C1 esterase deficiency (see *Rheumatology and clinical immunology*, Section 1.7).

Examination

The important things to check are:
- airway, tongue, lips
- respiratory: rate, effort, peak expiratory flow rate and O_2 saturation
- cardiovascular: heart rate and blood pressure
- rash.

Further management

For severe or recurrent reactions and for patients with asthma, give hydrocortisone 100–500 mg intravenously. If the patient remains in shock despite immediate therapy, commence rapid intravenous fluids. Remember that treatment may need to be continued for several hours following ingestion of an allergen or after an insect bite.

Prevention of further episodes

Anyone who has survived a life-threatening attack of anaphylaxis deserves specialist assessment to:
- determine precisely what they are allergic to
- receive advice about how to avoid further attacks, and how to respond if they occur, including instruction on the use of self-administered epinephrine (adrenaline—Epipen).

All such patients should be advised to wear a Medic Alert bracelet.

 See *Rheumatology and clinical immunology*, Sections 1.7, 1.9 and 2.2.
Project Team of the Resuscitation Council (UK). The emergency medical treatment of anaphylactic reactions. *J Accid Emerg Med* 1999; 16: 243–247.

2 Diseases and treatments

2.1 Overdoses

Aetiology

Overdoses may be the result of accidental overdosage of a prescribed or over-the-counter drug, social misuse or deliberate self-harm.

> Poisons and medicines are oftentimes the same substance given with different intents.
> (Peter Mere Latham, 1789–1875)

Clinical presentation

It is important to establish:
• What has been taken and when?
• Have any other tablets or alcohol been taken? (Always presume that they have.)
• Have there been previous episodes of self-harm?
• Past medical and psychiatric history, medications and allergies.
• Drug/alcohol abuse.
• Assess intent.

Physical signs

Priorities from the clinical examination include:
• Airway, breathing, circulation.
• Vital signs—temperature, pulse and respiration.
• Cardiovascular—is the patient shocked?
• Respiratory—is respiration adequate? Has the patient aspirated?
• GCS, neurological signs, possible brain-stem signs, pupillary size and reaction and a mental state examination.
• Temperature.

Investigations

Key tests include:
• BM stix.
• FBC, electrolytes, glucose, renal and liver function and clotting screen.
• Specific drug levels—aspirin and paracetamol levels should be performed 4 h after ingestion. Always presume a mixed overdose has been taken.

Table 31 Telephone numbers for Poisons Information Services.

City	Telephone number
Belfast	(028) 9024 0503
Birmingham	(0121) 507 5588/5589
Cardiff	(029) 2070 9901
Dublin	(00 353) 1837 9964/9966
Edinburgh	(0131) 536 2300
London	(020) 7635 9191
Newcastle	(0191) 282 0300

• ECG.
• Urine and serum samples may need to be saved for later toxicological analysis.
• Arterial blood gases (ABGs) if very unwell, carbon monoxide exposure, GCS of less than 10 or if ventilation is clinically inadequate.

 Advice should always be sought from the local Poisons Centre (Table 31).

Differential diagnosis

Poisoning should be considered in any patient presenting with altered consciousness or with unusual symptoms or signs.

Treatment

Patients who have taken an overdose range from those who walk into the department to those who are unconscious with cardiorespiratory collapse.

Assess ABC and resuscitate if very unwell, necessary.

If the patient looks unwell, give 100% O_2 and obtain intravenous access.

Immediate therapy

Specific treatments which take immediate priority are:
• If the BM stix estimation of blood sugar is low, give 50 mL 50% dextrose i.v. stat and continue with 10% dextrose by infusion until the BM is normal and stable.
• If the patient is hypothermic, start rewarming.
• If the pupils are small or there are signs of intravenous drug abuse, give 400 µg naloxone i.v. The dose may need to be repeated and, occasionally, an infusion of the drug will be needed.

Gastric decontamination, drug elimination

Activated charcoal

This is now the preferred method of gut decontamination if the dose of toxin taken is likely to cause moderate to severe toxicity. The single dose (50 g for adults) can be given up to 1 h after ingestion. However, certain drugs are not readily adsorbed to charcoal:

- iron salts
- lithium
- ethanol/methanol/ethylene glycol
- acids/alkalis
- organic solvents
- mercury
- lead
- fluorides
- potassium salts.

Multiple doses of charcoal should be considered for certain toxins:

- slow-release preparations
- carbamazepine
- dapsone
- digoxin
- paraquat
- phenobarbitone
- quinine
- Amanita phalloides (death cap mushroom).

 Charcoal is dangerous if aspirated.

Whole-bowel irrigation

Polyethylene glycol solution can be given orally or through a nasogastric tube until clear fluid appears per rectum. It can be used in ingestion of the following:

- slow-release preparations
- lithium
- iron
- arsenic
- lead oxide
- zinc sulphate.

It is contraindicated if there is:

- an inability to maintain the airway
- ileus
- bowel obstruction
- haemodynamic instability.

Gastric lavage

This technique is now rarely used and recent studies suggest that it does not improve clinical outcome. If it is to have any chance of success, it should be performed within 1 h of ingestion. There is some evidence that lavage can push ingested material through the pylorus, thereby speeding its absorption.

Contraindications to lavage are:

- inability to maintain the airway
- ingestion of corrosives
- ingestion of organic solvents.

Emetics

These are rarely used. There is no evidence that outcome is altered and it is difficult to give charcoal subsequently.

Haemodialysis

Haemodialysis is used for severe toxicity associated with:

- salicylates
- phenobarbital
- methanol
- ethylene glycol
- lithium.

Haemoperfusion

Haemoperfusion is useful for severe poisoning with:

- barbiturates
- chloral hydrate
- meprobamate
- theophylline.

Management of specific drug overdose

Paracetamol

Clinical details

- Nausea and vomiting may be the only early features.
- Right subcostal pain and tenderness suggest hepatic necrosis.

Ingestion may progress to acute liver failure.

 Paracetamol poisoning is a cause of lactic acidosis (see Section 1.19, p. 62).

Treatment

EARLY PRESENTATION

If a patient presents within 8 h of ingestion:

- Gastric decontamination; give activated charcoal if >150 mg/kg of paracetamol has been ingested in the last hour.

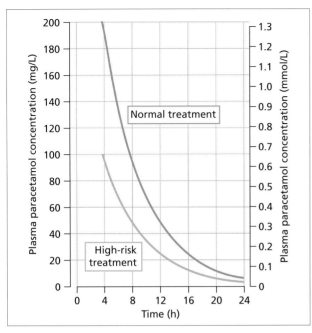

Fig. 44 Paracetamol treatment lines.

- Check aspirin and paracetamol levels at 4 h postingestion (as well as routine blood tests in overdose indicated above).
- The need for paracetamol antidotes may be assessed by plotting the 4-h plasma paracetamol level on a reference treatment curve (Fig. 44). Patients who are asymptomatic and have levels below the normal treatment line may be discharged (unless they require admission for psychiatric reasons).
- Antidotes—*N*-acetyl cysteine (NAC) is effective up to and possibly beyond 24 h postingestion. It is given intravenously in the UK and orally in the USA.
- For those receiving treatment, the INR, U & Es, and LFTs should be checked on completing the infusion and before discharge.
- All patients should be advised to return if vomiting or abdominal pain occur.
- Methionine 2.5 g orally can be given to those who are intolerant of NAC. It is protective if given within 12 h.

The intravenous dosage of NAC is:
- 150 mg/kg in 200 mL 5% dextrose over 15 min; then
- 50 mg/kg in 500 mL 5% dextrose over 4 h; then
- 100 mg/kg in 1000 mL 5% dextrose over 16 h.

- Patients on enzyme-inducing drugs (carbamazepine, phenytoin, rifampicin, phenobarbital) or who are malnourished (anorexia, HIV) may develop toxicity at much lower plasma paracetamol concentrations. Such patients should be treated if the 4-h level exceeds the high-risk treatment line (Fig. 44).
- Patients who drink >21 units of alcohol/week if male, or >14 units/week if female, may also be at greater risk.
- If the paracetamol level is unavailable within 8 h of ingestion and >150 mg/kg paracetamol has been taken, the antidote should be started and then stopped if the level is found to be below the treatment line.

Adverse reactions to NAC
- Nausea, flushing, urticaria, angioedema, bronchospasm and hypotension may occur.
- Reactions usually occur early and often resolve if NAC is stopped and intravenous chlorpheniramine given. The infusion may then be restarted at the lowest rate.

LATE PRESENTATION

Management of patients presenting 8–24 h postingestion:
- Check paracetamol/salicylate levels (as well as routine blood tests in overdose indicated above).
- If a significant amount has been taken (>150 mg/kg), start NAC.
- Continue NAC if levels are above treatment line or if alanine transferase (ALT), clotting or renal function are abnormal.
- At the end of treatment, the INR, U & E and LFTs should be checked. If these are normal and the patient is asymptomatic they may be considered for discharge.
- Patients should be advised to return if vomiting or abdominal pain occur.

The prognostic accuracy of the treatment nomogram is less certain if 15 h have elapsed since ingestion.

VERY LATE PRESENTATION

Management of patients presenting >24 h postingestion:
- Check paracetamol/salicylate levels (as well as routine blood tests in overdose indicated above).
- Those with abnormal clotting or renal function or with significant derangement of their LFTs need admission.
- Discuss with Poisons Centre.

Plasma paracetamol levels are hard to interpret if the paracetamol has been taken over a period of hours. Patients should be considered for treatment with NAC.

Salicylates

Clinical details

The important clinical features are hyperventilation, tinnitus, deafness, sweating, vasodilatation, convulsions, coma and death.

Management

Important aspects are:
- Gastric decontamination (see above).

• Check aspirin and paracetamol levels at 4 h postingestion (as well as routine blood tests in overdose indicated above).
• Check arterial blood gases.
If salicylate levels:
• >500 mg/L (3.6 mmol/L) consider alkaline diuresis with 1.26% $NaHCO_3$.
• >700 mg/L (5.1 mmol/L) consider haemodialysis.

Tricyclics

Clinical details

Coma, convulsions and dysrhythmias are the most serious signs of toxicity.

Tachycardia and QRS prolongation (>100 ms) on the ECG are also very worrying.

There may be symptoms related to:
• anticholinergic effects—blurred vision, dry mouth, pupillary dilation and urinary retention
• central effects—confusion, drowsiness, nystagmus, ataxia, hyperreflexia and hyperthermia.

TREATMENT

Important aspects are:
• Gastric decontamination (see above).
• Check aspirin and paracetamol levels at 4 h postingestion (as well as routine blood tests in overdose indicated above).
• Cardiac monitor.
• Intravenous diazepam for convulsions.
• Alkalinization with $NaHCO_3$ is indicated if there is systemic acidosis, prolonged QRS, ventricular dysrhythmias, hypotension or cardiac arrest. Aim for pH between 7.45 and 7.55.

• Dysrhythmias may respond to correction of hypoxia and acidosis.
• Antiarrhythmic drugs may be necessary but some can exacerbate the toxic effects of tricyclics (seek expert advice).

Opiates

Clinical details

Reduced consciousness, respiratory depression and pinpoint pupils are the classical clinical findings.

Treatment

Important aspects are:
• Give 100% O_2 and obtain intravenous access.
• Check BM and temperature.
• Give 400 μg naloxone i.v. and repeat as necessary.
• Always check levels of other drugs (for instance, paracetamol if co-proxamol has been taken).

• The half lives of most opiates are longer than naloxone. Repeated administration or an infusion of naloxone may be needed.
• Naloxone can be given via the endotracheal tube, intramuscularly or intraosseously if intravenous access cannot be obtained.
• Failure to respond promptly to naloxone should stimulate the search for other causes of reduced consciousness (see Section 1.26, p. 75).
• Illicit opiates are often cut with other toxic substances.

Jones AL, Volans G. Management of self-poisoning. *BMJ* 1999; 319: 1414–1417.

3 Investigations and practical procedures

3.1 Femoral vein cannulation

Aim

Insertion of a long catheter into the femoral vein is an alternative to internal jugular or subclavian vein cannulation. Practically, this procedure is often easier to perform and does not carry the risk of pneumothorax. It also allows another doctor unhindered access to the head and neck, e.g. for airway management. Measurement of the CVP, however, is less accurate than with internal jugular or subclavian vein cannulation.

Indications

These include:
- infusion of fluids
- infusion of drugs
- measurement of the CVP when internal jugular or subclavian vein cannulation is not possible or desirable
- insertion of pacing wire
- access for haemodialysis/haemofiltration.

Contraindications

These include:
- venous thrombosis in the femoral or iliac veins
- trauma to the femoral area or pelvis.

Patient information

If the patient is conscious, tell them what you are going to do and maintain their dignity as much as possible.

Practical details

Preparation

Patient

It is ideal to know the patient's clotting and platelet count. However, patients who require this procedure are often seriously ill, in which case do not delay waiting for results. If the patient is ill enough to require a femoral line they should be on O_2, a pulse oximeter and a cardiac monitor.

Personnel

A nurse should be present to help you with strict aseptic technique and to monitor the patient throughout the procedure.

Equipment

Make sure you have everything on the trolley before you start:
- Dressing pack, drapes and gloves, all sterile.
- Local anaesthetic, syringe and needle.
- Seldinger catheter set with 5 mL syringe, introducer needle, guidewire, dilator and central line, or 16G long cannula
- Saline or Hepsal flush
- Three-way tap (×3 if triple lumen catheter)
- Small scalpel blade, silk suture and sterile occlusive dressing.

Technique

1 Identify your landmarks (Fig. 45). The femoral vein lies directly medial to the femoral artery in the femoral triangle.
2 Clean and drape the skin.
3 Infiltrate the skin and subcutaneous tissue with 1% lidocaine (lignocaine).
4 Flush the lumen(s) of the central line with saline or

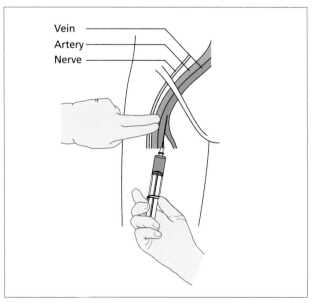

Vein
Artery
Nerve

Fig. 45 Femoral vein cannulation.

Hepsal and ensure you have all your equipment within easy reach.

5 Feel the femoral pulse and insert the introducer needle one finger breadth medial to this, angulating it slightly towards the patient's head, but keeping it in line with the long axis of the leg. Advance slowly, aspirating all the time until there is free flow of blood into the syringe.

6 Insert a cannula-over-needle directly or—if using the Seldinger technique—proceed as follows.

 It may be helpful to remember 'NAVY': nerve, artery, vein, Y-fronts, when locating the position of the femoral vein.

Seldinger technique

This technique, which is more reliable than cannula-over-needle techniques, is widely used for arterial or venous cannulation:

• Once you are in the vein and can aspirate blood freely, remove the syringe and occlude the end of the needle with your finger to prevent air embolism.

• Pass the guidewire into the vein ensuring it passes freely. If there is any resistance then remove the wire and check that blood can still be aspirated easily, then try again.

• Remove the needle, leaving the wire in the vein.

• Nick the skin at the base of the wire with the small scalpel blade to allow easy passage of the dilator. Pass the dilator over the wire through the subcutaneous tissue and then remove it, leaving the wire *in situ*.

• Pass the central line over the wire into the vein. Remove the wire and check that you can aspirate blood freely through the cannula.

With the line in place, flush with saline or Hepsal and close the line off to air. Secure with a suture and place a sterile occlusive dressing over the site.

 Make sure that you can always see the end of the guidewire. Never let it disappear entirely into the cannula—it has been known for the wire to be lost in the vein, necessitating surgical removal.
Problem: the dilator will not pass over the guidewire without difficulty.
Answer: do not push it hard! If you do, you will crimp the guidewire and will have to remove both dilator and wire.
• Remove dilator and check that the wire moves freely in the vessel (advance and retract a few centimetres).
• Check that the skin has been properly nicked with a scalpel (a small tag is often responsible for difficulty).
• Try to advance the dilator again—rotating the dilator as you push sometimes helps.

After the procedure

Organize an abdominal radiograph to identify the position of the catheter.

Complications

Major complications

These include:
• infection
• damage to the femoral nerve
• arteriovenous fistula formation
• thrombosis of the femoral or iliac vein
• lost catheters.

Minor complications

These include:
• haematoma formation
• arterial puncture
• localized infection
• misplacement of the catheter.

3.2 Central vein cannulation

Aim

Insertion of a long cannula into the internal jugular vein or subclavian vein. Either a cannula-over-needle or Seldinger (guidewire-through-needle) technique may be used; the latter is to be preferred.

Indications

These include:
• measurement of CVP
• administration of some drugs, e.g. dopamine
• parenteral feeding
• insertion of pulmonary artery catheter, temporary cardiac pacing wire or haemodialysis/haemofiltration catheter
• infusion of fluids in the severely ill.

Contraindications

There are no absolute contraindications but relative contraindications are:
• abnormal clotting
• severe respiratory disease—where pneumothorax may precipitate respiratory failure
• marked hypovolaemia, when the technique is difficult, time-consuming and carries more risk of complications. It is always best to correct hypovolaemia through large-bore peripheral or femoral vein access before inserting a central vein cannula.

Patient information

The patient may be too ill to give informed consent. If they are conscious and alert, explain what you are about to do and emphasize the need to remain still during the procedure.

Practical details

Preparation

Patient

Ideally, the patient's clotting should be checked first, however, in sick patients in whom close haemodynamic monitoring or fluid or drug administration is urgent, do not delay. The patient should be on a cardiac monitor and pulse oximeter.

Personnel

A nurse should be present to help you with strict aseptic technique and to observe the cardiac monitor, pulse oximeter and the patient during the procedure.

Equipment

Make sure you have everything on the trolley before you start. The equipment list is identical to that for femoral vein cannulation.

Technique

Internal jugular vein cannulation using the Seldinger technique

1 Lie the patient down, preferably with head-down tilt, and turn their head away from the side you intend to cannulate.
2 Identify your landmarks (Fig. 46). The internal jugular vein lies superficial, lateral and parallel to the carotid artery. Identify the apex of the triangle formed by the two heads of the sternocleidomastoid muscle at the level of the thyroid cartilage. This is where you will introduce the needle—one of the so-called 'high approaches' that minimize the risk of pneumothorax.
3 Clean and drape the skin.
4 Infiltrate the skin and subcutaneous tissue with 1% lidocaine (lignocaine).
5 Flush the lumen(s) of the central line with saline or Hepsal, and ensure you have all your equipment within easy reach.
6 Attach the introducer needle to the 5 mL syringe and, keeping one finger on the carotid pulse, insert the needle just lateral to this at 45° to the skin. Aim for the ipsilateral nipple in men or the anterior superior iliac spine in

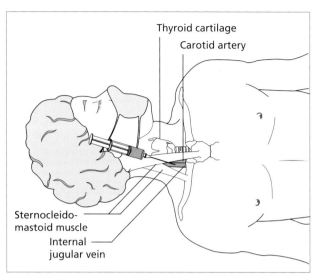

Fig. 46 Internal jugular vein cannulation.

women. Advance the needle slowly whilst aspirating for blood. You will only need to insert it a few centimetres as the vein lies superficially. If you do not hit the vein, withdraw the needle to just below the skin and aim slightly more medially and superficially.
7 Once you are in the vein and can aspirate blood freely, remove the syringe and occlude the end of the needle with your finger (to prevent air embolism). Proceed with the Seldinger technique (see Section 3.1, p. 87).

With the line in place, flush with saline or Hepsal and close the line off to air. Secure with a suture and place a sterile occlusive dressing over the site.

If measurement of the CVP is needed, attach the manometer set to the patient and adjust the zero reference point on the manometer so it is at the level of the patient's right atrium (midaxillary line). Alternatively, an electronic transducer and oscilloscope may be used to continuously measure the CVP which also needs to be zeroed and calibrated prior to use.

Subclavian vein cannulation using the Seldinger technique

The axillary vein becomes the subclavian vein at the lateral border of the first rib and extends for 3–4 cm just deep to the clavicle. It forms the brachiocephalic vein with the internal jugular vein behind the sternoclavicular joint. The right subclavian vein is easier to cannulate than the left.
1 Identify the landmarks (Fig. 47). Locate the suprasternal notch, sternoclavicular joint and acromioclavicular joint and select a point one finger-breadth below the junction of the medial third and middle third of the clavicle.
2 Clean and drape the skin.
3 Infiltrate the skin and subcutaneous tissue with 1% lidocaine (lignocaine).

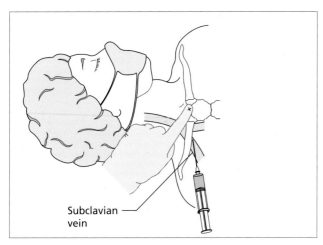

Subclavian
vein

Fig. 47 Subclavian vein cannulation.

4 Flush the lumen(s) of the central line with saline or Hepsal, and ensure you have all your equipment within easy reach.

5 Insert the introducer needle attached to the 5 mL syringe until it hits the clavicle and 'walk' the tip down the clavicle until it is lying just under the inferior border. Advance the needle, aspirating for blood, towards the contralateral sternoclavicular joint. Try to keep the track of the needle parallel to the bed in order to avoid puncturing the pleura or subclavian artery.

6 Once blood is aspirated freely, rotate the bevel of the needle towards the heart in order to maximize the chance of the wire passing down the brachiocephalic vein rather than up the internal jugular vein.

7 Insert the central line using the Seldinger technique.

After the procedure

Arrange a chest radiograph to exclude pneumothorax and to confirm the correct position of the catheter. The tip should ideally lie in the superior vena cava just above the right atrium.

 Do not infuse a large amount of fluid until the catheter is confirmed as being correctly sited.

Complications

Major complications

These include:
- pneumothorax
- haemopneumothorax
- nerve damage
- chylothorax (particularly with left subclavian lines due to damage to the thoracic duct)
- infection
- arteriovenous fistula
- venous thrombosis
- lost catheters
- erosion of superior vena cava or even the wall of the right atrium by the catheter.

 In ventilated patients even a small pneumothorax must be treated with a chest drain as it may rapidly turn into a tension pneumothorax.

Minor complications

These include:
- arterial puncture. If the carotid artery is inadvertently punctured, apply pressure and then reattempt
- ventricular asystoles—withdraw the cannula slightly
- localized infection or phlebitis
- misplacement of the cannula. This should be recognized on the chest radiograph. Reposition as necessary
- haematoma formation

 If the carotid artery is punctured and forms a haematoma on one side do not attempt internal jugular vein cannulation on the other side, especially in patients with abnormal clotting, as this may result in airway compromise if bilateral haematomas occur. Cannulate the subclavian or femoral vein instead.

 Interpretation of results

The CVP does give an indication of the patient's blood volume but is also affected by the contractile state of the myocardium, venous tone, intrathoracic pressure and pulmonary arterial pressure.

The CVP does not always provide accurate information on left-sided cardiac filling pressures. These can be low even though the CVP is normal or high, the classic example of this being severe PE.

Before measuring the CVP make sure that the system has been zeroed to the midaxillary reference point and that the venous pressure swings with respiration.

Table 32 lists the common causes of an abnormal CVP.

Table 32 Causes of an abnormal central venous pressure (CVP).

Raised CVP	Low CVP
Fluid overload	Hypovolaemia
Right ventricular failure, e.g. right ventricular infarction	Septic shock
Massive pulmonary embolism	Anaphylactic
Cardiac tamponade	shock
Tension pneumothorax	
Blocked catheter—causes a sustained high reading with a damped waveform	
Infusion of fluid, e.g. through an infusion pump at the same time the pressure is being measured	
Catheter tip in right ventricle will give an unexpectedly high pressure	

3.3 Intercostal chest drain insertion

Aim

Insertion of a drain connected to an underwater seal into the thoracic cavity to remove air, fluid and/or blood.

Indications

These include the treatment of:
- large or symptomatic spontaneous pneumothorax [1]
- traumatic pneumothorax
- haemothorax
- empyema.

Tension pneumothorax

Never wait for a chest radiograph if a tension pneumothorax has been diagnosed clinically and the patient is in haemodynamic and/or respiratory distress.

Do an immediate needle thoracocentesis and then insert a chest drain.

How to perform needle thoracocentesis

Simply insert a 20G cannula into the second intercostal space in the midclavicular line.

If a tension pneumothorax is present you will hear a sudden rush of air when the cap is removed from the cannula as it enters the parietal pleura.

This technique can also be used to aspirate a small pneumothorax, in which case the area should be anaesthetized first and the cannula connected to a 3-way tap and a 60 mL syringe.

Bullae

Take care not to insert a chest drain into an emphysematous bulla mistakenly diagnosed on the chest radiograph as a pneumothorax.

Patient information

If the patient is conscious, tell them what you are going to do and why. Explain that you will give them some local anaesthetic but that they will feel some discomfort. Impress upon them the need to remain still throughout the procedure.

Practical details

Preparation

Patient

1 Arrange a chest radiograph to confirm the diagnosis and to exclude the presence of an emphysematous bulla.
2 If the procedure is being done for a haemothorax make sure that you have two large-bore intravenous cannulas in place first and blood available for transfusion.
3 Consider administering a small dose of diamorphine before the procedure and have more of the drug available if needed as the procedure is undertaken.
4 Put the patient on O_2 and monitor pulse oximetry and ECG.

Personnel

Make sure you have a nurse with you to help you with strict aseptic technique and to monitor the patient.

Equipment

Make sure you have everything on the trolley before you start:
- basic sterile pack and other equipment
- local anaesthetic and a syringe with orange and green needles for infiltration
- 28 Ch chest drain (larger if a haemothorax is present)
- scalpel blade and handle
- Spencer Wells forceps
- needle holder
- curved scissors
- suture scissors
- tissue forceps
- 1/0 or 2/0 silk suture
- two 3/0 monofilament sutures
- dressings and adhesives
- underwater seal bottle with connections.

Technique

1 Position the patient. If possible have them semi-recumbent with their hand resting behind their head.
2 Identify your landmarks (Fig. 48). The safest position for an intercostal drain is in the fifth intercostal space in the midaxillary line.
3 Clean and drape the skin.
4 Infiltrate the skin with local anaesthetic using the orange needle and then infiltrate down to the pleura using the green needle.
5 Make a 2–3 cm incision through the skin and subcutaneous adipose tissue along the line of the intercostal space just above the edge of the lower rib.

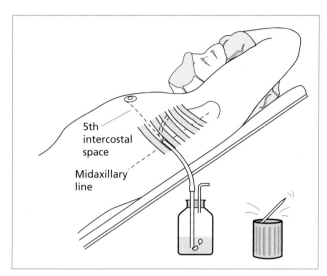

Fig. 48 Intercostal drain insertion.

6 Bluntly dissect down to the pleura using the Spencer Wells forceps.

7 Puncture the parietal pleura with the tip of the forceps and then insert your finger to enlarge the hole. Sweep your finger around to clear any adhesions or clots. Make sure that there is adequate space to insert the chest drain without using force.

8 Remove any trochar from the intercostal drain and slide the drain over your finger into the thoracic cavity. If it is in the correct position you will see 'fogging' of the tube.

9 Connect the drain to the underwater seal and confirm correct placement by ensuring that the fluid level is swinging with respiration.

10 Insert a 3/0 monfilament suture at 90° to the line of the skin incision at the site of the chest drain, but do not tie it. This will be used to close the skin after the drain is removed.

11 Secure the tube with the 1/0 or 2/0 silk. Tie it so that the skin is closed either side of the drain and then wrap it around and tie it to the drain as many times as its length allows.

12 If the incision is gaping close the skin either side of the drain with another 3/0 monofilament.

13 Place a gauze dressing around the site and secure with 'Mefix' or similar. Wrap a tongue of tape around the tube for security.

Chest drains—how to find the fifth intercostal space

- In someone without breasts the fifth intercostal space is usually at the level of the nipple.
- If a person has large breasts then the position of the fifth intercostal space corresponds to the lower border of the patient's contralateral hand when this is placed flat against the chest wall with the thumb in the axilla.

Chest drains—making the incision

Avoid making the incision just below the upper rib as this may cause damage to the intercostal nerves and vessels which lie underneath the lower edge of the rib.

Chest drains—use of the trochar

The only place for a trochar is in the bin. If used to insert the chest drain it can cause serious damage.

Chest drains—closing the hole

Do not use a purse-string suture as this produces unsightly scars and is unnecessary.

After the procedure

Immediate

Get a chest radiograph to confirm correct positioning of the tube and ensure that the fluid level in the tube is swinging with respiration once it has been secured. It is vital to prescribe adequate analgesia.

Subsequently

A daily chest radiograph is indicated to ensure correct siting of the tube and adequate resolution of the pneumothorax, haemothorax or empyema.

Remove the tube when the radiograph shows full resolution and the tube is no longer bubbling when the patient coughs. Repeat the chest radiograph after tube removal.

Chest drain tubes

Never clamp the tube; this is unnecessary and can lead to a tension pneumothorax.

Complications

Major complications

Major complications include:
- Damage to intrathoracic and/or abdominal organs or vessels. This can be obviated by using the finger sweep and never using the trochar.
- Damage to the intercostal nerve, artery or vein, which may result in intercostal neuralgia or conversion of a pneumothorax to a haemothorax.
- Introduction of pleural infection, perhaps with subsequent empyema formation.
- Pulmonary oedema. This is a possibility if the lung expands too rapidly.
- Surgical emphysema. If this develops, insert a new tube.

Minor complications

Minor complications include localized cellulitis and localized haematoma formation.

Persistent pneumothorax?

Consider:
• Large primary leak.
• Leakage at the skin or underwater seal.
• Plugged bronchus.
• Bronchopleural fistula.

Failure of fluid level to swing with respiration?

Consider:
• Is the tube kinked? Try loosening the dressing or withdrawing the tube slightly.
• Is the tube blocked?
• Is the tube in the wrong position?

1 Miller AC, Harvey JE on behalf of Standards of Care Committee. British Thoracic Society guidelines for the management of spontaneous pneumothorax. *BMJ* 1993; 307: 114–116. (This is soon to be updated.)

3.4 Arterial blood gases

Aim

To measure arterial P_{O_2}, P_{CO_2} and pH.

Indications

These include pulse oximetry showing P_{O_2} <95% and any acute unexplained severe illness.

Contraindications

There are no absolute contraindications. Severe bleeding disorder is a relative contraindication.

Patient information

Explain the procedure to the patient (patients who have had ABGs performed know just how painful they can be).

Practical details

Preparation

Patient

Choose the site for arterial puncture carefully.
• Radial. First, perform the Allen test to check patency of the ulnar artery. Ask the patient to clench their fist firmly. Apply pressure to the radial artery. On relaxing the fist, the hand should pink up within 10 s.
• Femoral.
• Brachial.

Equipment

Before taking the sample, ensure you know where the blood gas machine is and how to use it! You will need:
• A preheparinized arterial blood gas syringe (or 2 mL syringe into which you have drawn up and then expelled 0.5 mL of 5000 U/mL heparin).
• 18/23/25G needles.
• Alcohol swabs.

Technique

1 Glove up.
2 Lay the index and middle fingers of your non-dominant hand along the line of the artery as a guide (Fig. 49).
3 For radial and brachial samples, hold the syringe at 45–60° to the skin and slowly advance in the line of the artery. For femoral samples, hold the syringe at 90° to the skin.
4 A flush of blood indicates puncture of a vessel. With some ABG syringes, the arterial pressure will fill the syringe to a predetermined volume. In others you will need to aspirate 1–2 mL.

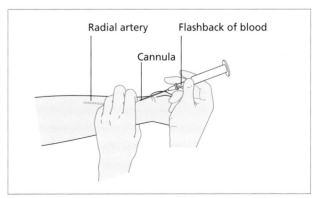

Fig. 49 Radial artery blood gases. The artery should be palpated and two fingers placed along the line of the artery. The needle should be inserted at 45–60° to the skin and slowly advanced in the direction of the artery. A flashback of blood indicates successful puncture.

5 Apply pressure to the puncture site for 3 min (5 min if the patient is anticoagulated).
6 Expel all air from the syringe. Remove and dispose of the needle and cap the syringe. If there is to be a delay in processing the sample, pack it in ice.

 25G needles are perfectly adequate to obtain ABG samples from a radial artery. 18G or 23G are needed for a femoral sample.
There is debate over the use of lidocaine (lignocaine). Whilst undoubtedly useful at easing pain if you are unlucky enough to fail first time, its use is painful in itself and often makes palpation of the artery more difficult.

After the procedure

Check that bleeding has stopped.

Complications

The main complication is haematoma.

Interpretation of arterial blood gases

Table 33 shows normal arterial blood gas values. Look at the following in the order shown below.

pH

Consider Fig. 50. If pH <7.35, the patient is acidotic. If pH >7.45, the patient is alkalotic. A value between 7.35 and 7.45 is normal, but could be obtained because the patient is compensating: primary metabolic disturbance with secondary respiratory compensation; or primary respiratory disturbance with secondary metabolic compensation.

P_{CO_2}

Elevated (>6 kPa)

This is almost certainly respiratory acidosis, when the primary abnormality is elevation of P_{CO_2} due to alveolar hypoventilation. The body attempts to compensate by retaining HCO_3^-. However, conservation of HCO_3^- by

Table 33 Normal arterial blood gas values.

Arterial blood gas	Value
pH	7.35–7.45
P_{CO_2}	4.5–6.0 kPa
HCO_3	22–28 mmol/L
SBE	±2 mmol/L
P_{O_2}	10.5–14 kPa
O_2 saturation	95–100%

SBE, standard base excess.

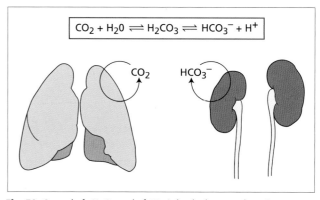

Fig. 50 Control of pH. Control of CO_2 is by the lungs and respiratory centre. The kidneys play the major role in maintaining the HCO_3^- concentration.

the kidneys takes time and the associated elevation of HCO_3^- (secondary metabolic alkalosis) suggests that the respiratory acidosis is chronic.
A slight increase in P_{CO_2} can occur as a respiratory compensation for metabolic alkalosis.

Reduced (<4.5 kPa)

There are two possibilities: metabolic acidosis and respiratory alkalosis.

Metabolic acidosis

The primary abnormality in metabolic acidosis is a reduction in HCO_3^-. The body compensates by losing CO_2 through the lungs: secondary respiratory alkalosis. This is one of the mechanisms driving hyperventilation on exercise; when you exercise and increase lactate production, you breathe quicker to remove CO_2.

Respiratory alkalosis

The primary abnormality in respiratory alkalosis is loss of CO_2 as a consequence of overbreathing. The body compensates by losing HCO_3^- in the kidney (secondary metabolic acidosis).

HCO_3^-

Elevated (>28 mmol/L)

This usually occurs as compensation for chronic respiratory acidosis (see above). In metabolic alkalosis, the primary abnormality is a rise in HCO_3^-. There is little, if any, compensatory rise in P_{CO_2}.

Reduced (<22 mmol/L)

This is the primary abnormality in metabolic acidosis (see

above). Reduced HCO_3^- also occurs as compensation for the reduced P_{CO_2} of respiratory alkalosis.

Standard base excess (normal ±2 mmol/L)

The standard base excess (SBE) is a figure calculated by many blood gas machines as an aid to data interpretation. The principles of the calculation are as follows:
• Predict the pH that would arise in normal blood in the presence of the P_{CO_2} actually measured. If the P_{CO_2} is high, then the predicted pH is low; if the P_{CO_2} is low, then the predicted pH is high.
• Calculate the amount of acid or base that would have to be added to the blood to change the calculated pH into the pH as actually measured.
• This is the base deficit or excess, in mmol/L, which quantifies the metabolic component of acid–base disturbance. The more negative the value for SBE, the greater the degree of acidosis.

P_{O_2} *and* O_2 *saturation*

Are the measurements low, normal or high for that patient? Many patients with chronic lung or heart disease have a P_{O_2} of 7–8 kPa and are quite happy!

See *Respiratory medicine*, Section 3.6.1.
Adrogué HJ, Madias NE. Management of life-threatening acid-base disorders. First of two parts. *N Engl J Med* 1998; 338: 26–34.
Adrogué HJ, Madias NE. Management of life-threatening acid-base disorders. Second of two parts. *N Engl J Med* 1998; 338: 107–111.

3.5 Lumbar puncture

Aim

To remove CSF for diagnostic or therapeutic purposes.

Indications

Diagnostic indications are:
• meningitis
• subarachnoid haemorrhage
• intrathecal malignancy.
    Therapeutic indications include:
• intrathecal drug administration
• benign intracranial hypertension.

Contraindications

Contraindications include:
• raised intracranial pressure
• posterior fossa or spinal cord mass lesion
• local sepsis
• bleeding tendency.

Lumbar puncture and risk of coning

If the patient is unconscious, drowsy, has clinical features of raised intracranial pressure or focal neurological signs, a CT scan must be performed prior to lumbar puncture.
    If there is likely to be a delay and meningitis is a diagnostic possibility, antibiotic treatment should be started immediately.

Practical details

Preparation

Equipment

Ensure that you have the necessary equipment:
• sterile gown, gloves and drapes
• antiseptic
• 5–10 mL 1% lidocaine (lignocaine) with 25G and 18G needles
• lumbar puncture (LP) needles and sterile manometer
• serum glucose bottle, three sterile 20 mL containers (labelled 1, 2, 3)
• dressing pack.

Patient

Explain the procedure carefully to the patient.

Technique

1 Ask the patient to lie on the bed (Fig. 51a). Positioning is all-important: the knees should be drawn up towards the chest to open the space between the spinous processes and the spine should be parallel to the bed.
2 Gown and glove up.
3 Prepare the skin with antiseptic and cover with sterile drapes.
4 Locate the puncture site (L3/L4 or L4/L5). Anaesthetize the skin and subcutaneous tissues with approximately 5 mL 1% lidocaine (lignocaine) using the 25G needle. Switch to the 18G needle and infiltrate the deeper tissues.
5 Assemble the manometer. Unscrew the tops of the sterile containers.
6 Insert the LP needle at 90° to the skin. Advance slowly, aiming between two spinous processes. As the needle enters the dural space, there is a slight loss of resistance (Fig. 51b).

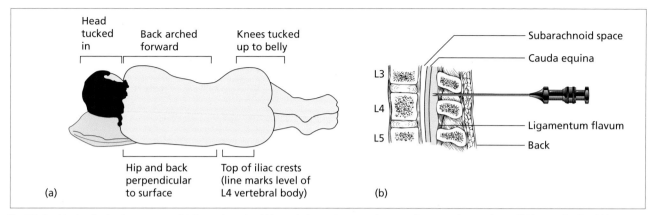

Fig. 51 Positioning for lumbar puncture. (a) The patient should be curled up to increase the space between the vertebrae. (b) The needle should be advanced slowly until it penetrates the ligamentum flavum. A flashback of CSF when the stylet is removed indicates correct positioning.

	Pressure (cm H$_2$O)	White cells (per μL)	Protein (g/L)	Glucose (mmol/L)
Normal	6–15	<5 Mononuclear cells	0.2–0.4	2.5–4.5
Bacterial meningitis	Normal or ↑	↑↑↑ Polymorphs	1–5	0.2–2.2
Viral meningitis	Normal or ↑	↑ to ↑↑ Lymphocytes	<1	(r)
Tumour	Normal or ↑	0–100s Mononuclear cells Malignant cells also possible	↑↑	(r) or ↓

Table 34 Cerebrospinal fluid findings in various conditions.

7 Remove the stylet and ensure that CSF drips freely from the needle. If it does not, insert the stylet and advance the needle a few millimetres, then check again.

8 Attach the manometer and measure the pressure (normal 6–15 cm water).

9 Collect CSF samples:
- 2–5 drops for biochemistry
- 5–10 drops for bacteriology (ask for urgent microscopy and Gram stain, culture, sensitivities and viral studies)
- 5–10 drops for cytology
- for SAH, the red cell count in consecutive samples can help to distinguish SAH from a bloody tap. The sample should also be examined for xanthochromia (oxyhaemoglobin and bilirubin).

10 Always send blood samples for glucose and protein estimation at the same time. The CSF glucose concentration is normally 60–80% of the blood level.

11 Remove the needle and dress the wound.

12 Ask the patient to remain lying flat for 2–4 h to reduce the severity of post-LP headache.

Lumbar puncture—problems

1 *Unable to obtain CSF?*
This is usually due to problems with positioning. Reposition the patient. Ensure you are advancing the needle at 90° to the back. Ask for help.

2 *Bloody tap?*
This is common, occurring in approximately 20% of cases. Measure the red cell count on three consecutive CSF samples and look for xanthochromia in order to distinguish between a traumatic tap and SAH.

Lumbar puncture—problems (*continued*)

3 *Post-LP headache?*
This too is common and may occur a day or two after the procedure. Seek advice if the headache is severe and unrelieved by simple analgesia.

After the procedure

Table 34 is a guide to help you in interpreting the CSF findings.

3.6 Pacing

Aim

To artificially (electrically) stimulate cardiac contraction and thereby determine heart rate.

EXTERNAL PACING (Fig. 52)

Indications

Haemodynamically significant bradycardia that is unresponsive to atropine. It may be beneficial in ventricular standstill if instituted early but has not been proved to be of overall benefit for the treatment of asystole.

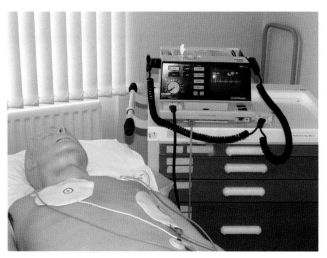

Fig. 52 External pacer. A modern monitor/defibrillator/external pacer.

External pacing

Ensure you know how to use the equipment and where it is stored. When it is needed there is no time to read the manual!

Practical details

Technique

1 One electrode should be placed in a position corresponding to lead V2–3 of the ECG. The other should be placed on the posterior of the chest below the left scapula (Fig. 52).

2 Ensure that the pacing box is set to demand (usually with a rate of 60 beats/min). Connect the leads to the patient and slowly increase the current. A current of 50–100 mA is usually required.

3 Ventricular capture is indicated when the pacing spike is associated with a ventricular complex and a palpable pulse wave.

4 Administer intravenous analgesia and/or sedation. Use of an external pacemaker is extremely uncomfortable.

5 Make immediate preparations for transvenous pacing. External pacing is unreliable and should be continued for as short a period as possible (<40 min).

Failure to capture with external pacing?

- Ensure the current is high enough.
- Seek immediate help.
- Try alternative electrodes or electrode positions.
- Pacing may be attempted by fist pacing (forceful, rhythmic thumping of the left anterior chest).
- Commence an isoprenaline infusion.

TEMPORARY TRANSVENOUS PACING

The procedure of temporary transvenous pacing is beyond the scope of this module. It should be learnt under supervision as it is now a semielective procedure.

It is important to understand the terminology used to describe pacemaker function and to be aware of reasons for failure of a temporary pacemaker. A pacemaker generator is shown in Fig. 53.

Terminology

Capture

The pacing stimulus generates contraction of the myocardium ('captures' it) and the ECG shows a pacing spike followed by a complex generated by the paced chamber. Commonly, it is the ventricle being paced and the QRS complex resembles a ventricular ectopic beat.

Threshold

This is the minimum output from the pacemaker generator that results in capture of the paced chamber.

Fixed vs demand pacing

Fixed pacing means that the pacemaker generates pacing stimuli at regular intervals regardless of any underlying cardiac rhythm. This mode is rarely used as competition with the underlying rhythm may generate dysrhythmias.

Demand pacing is used in most instances. The pacemaker senses the underlying cardiac rhythm and spontaneous

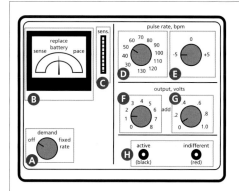

A Mode: demand vs fixed
B Pointer: allows you to see whether an intrinsic beat is sensed or if the patient is being paced
C Sensitivity should be set at 1.0
D Rate setting
E Rate adjustment by ± 5 bpm
F & G Voltage adjustment: should be set at 2 volts above threshold
H Lead terminals

Fig. 53 Pacemaker generator.

complexes inhibit output from the pacemaker. If a spontaneous complex does not occur within a set interval, the pacemaker generates a pacing stimulus.

Problems with transvenous pacing systems

Increasing threshold

Temporary transvenous pacemakers should have their threshold tested at least daily as this often increases over time. Threshold is tested by gradually turning down the pacemaker output until failure to capture occurs. The pacemaker output should be set at three times the threshold voltage or 3 V, whichever is the higher. Increasing threshold is an indication for repositioning of the wire or urgent permanent pacing (as appropriate).

Loss of electrical continuity

There are usually four connections between the electrodes of the pacing wire and the pacemaker generator. All four should be checked regularly as loss of continuity may result in syncope.

Electrode displacement

The tip of a temporary transvenous pacemaker is situated in the apex of the right ventricle. Migration of the pacing wire can lead to an increasing threshold without symptoms or sudden syncope.

If a patient with a transvenous pacemaker suddenly becomes symptomatic:
1 Check that the pacemaker generator is switched on.
2 Check lead connections.
3 Increase voltage to maximum.
4 If symptoms persist, substitute external pacing and call for help.

See *Cardiology*, Sections 2.2.1 and 3.5.
Morley-Davies A, Cobbe SM. Cardiac pacing. *Lancet* 1997; 349: 41–46.

3.7 Haemodynamic monitoring

Aim

To obtain measurements that give more information about circulatory function than can be gleaned from clinical examination and non-invasive techniques.

Clinical examination and non-invasive techniques

Capillary refill

A capillary refill time of >2 s indicates inadequate tissue perfusion. Capillary refill may be assessed by compression of the nail bed for 5 s. Pressure is then released and the time for capillary filling is measured. The extremity should be lifted slightly above the level of the heart to ensure that it is refilled by arteriolar and not venous capillaries.

Pulse volume

This is related to pulse pressure (the difference between systolic and diastolic pressures). In low output shock, the pulse pressure narrows making the pulse 'thready' and eventually impossible to feel.

Temperature

The skin to core temperature gradient provides semi-quantitative measurement of the degree of vasoconstriction. Change in the gradient over time indicates improvement or worsening of the clinical state.

Urine output

The kidneys receive approximately 25% of cardiac output. Glomerular filtration rate depends on renal perfusion. Hourly assessment of urine output provides a good measure of the adequacy of resuscitation (in adults this should exceed 0.5 mL/kg/h).

Haematocrit

Oxygen delivery to the tissues depends on the O_2 capacity of the blood and its viscocity. Optimal delivery occurs with an Hb around 10 g/dL.

ECG, blood pressure and pulse oximetry

Tissue O_2 delivery is dependent on arterial O_2 content (a function of arterial O_2 saturation and haemoglobin concentration) and cardiac output. Monitoring of heart rhythm, blood pressure and arterial O_2 saturation are basic aids to haemodynamic assessment.

Invasive techniques

Central venous pressure

CVP reflects venous return to the heart, right heart compliance, intrathoracic pressure and the position of

Table 35 Differential diagnosis of abnormal central venous pressure (CVP) readings.

CVP reading	Primary pathology	
High	Common	Biventricular failure
		Tricuspid regurgitation
		Pulmonary hypertension
		Fluid overload
		Artefact, e.g. catheter tip in right ventricle
	Consider	Cardiac tamponade
		Tension pneumothorax
		SVC obstruction
		Pulmonary stenosis
Low	Common	Hypovolaemia
		Septicaemia

SVC, superior vena cava.

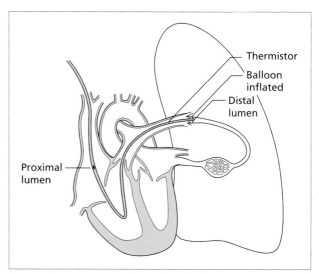

Fig. 54 Pulmonary artery catheter with the balloon wedged in a medium-sized artery. With the balloon inflated there is a column of blood from the tip of the catheter to the left atrium. Pulmonary artery wedge pressure usually reflects left atrial pressure. See text.

the patient. It is an indirect measure of the state of hydration.

Changes in CVP are a better guide than absolute values. Readings should be taken from a constant zero point using an anatomical landmark (for instance, the midaxillary line at the fourth intercostal space or the manubriosternal angle) with the patient in the same position in the bed.

Causes of abnormal CVP values are shown in Table 35.

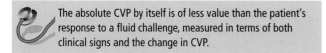

The absolute CVP by itself is of less value than the patient's response to a fluid challenge, measured in terms of both clinical signs and the change in CVP.

Intra-arterial blood pressure monitoring

Invasive monitoring of the arterial pressure allows beat-to-beat measurement of blood pressure and frequent assessment of arterial blood gases.

Pulmonary artery (flotation or Swan–Ganz) catheter

Pulmonary artery catheters are frequently used to monitor therapy for critically ill patients whose fluid and circulatory status is uncertain. A balloon-tipped, flow-directed catheter is inserted into a large vein (commonly the subclavian or internal jugular). As the catheter is advanced via the right atrium and ventricle into the pulmonary artery, pressure recordings of each chamber can be made.

Inflation of the balloon when the catheter is in a medium-sized pulmonary artery allows it to 'wedge' and occlude distal flow (Fig. 54). The pressure recorded at the tip (pulmonary capillary wedge pressure, PCWP) provides

Table 36 Conditions where PCWP does not reflect LVEDP.

PCWP > LVEDP	PCWP < LVEDP
Mitral stenosis	Severe LVF
↑ Intrathoracic pressure	
↑ Pulmonary vascular resistance	

LVEDP, left ventricular end-diastolic pressure; LVF, left ventricular failure; PCWP, pulmonary capillary wedge pressure.

an indirect measurement of the left atrial pressure, which in turn reflects left ventricular end-diastolic pressure (LVEDP) with certain provisos. Conditions where PCWP does not accurately reflect LVEDP are shown in Table 36.

Cardiac output can be estimated using thermodilution. A volume of saline at known temperature (usually 0°C) is injected via a proximal port of the catheter. The change in temperature at the tip of the catheter over time is measured and used to generate a thermal dilution curve, the area under the curve being inversely proportional to the cardiac output (with high cardiac output the saline is diluted in a large volume of warm blood; with low cardiac output it is diluted in a lesser volume).

Many other haemodynamic values can be obtained either directly or indirectly from pulmonary artery catheter measurements, e.g. cardiac index, systemic vascular resistance and pulmonary artery pressures.

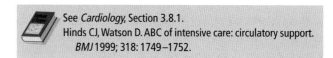

See *Cardiology*, Section 3.8.1.
Hinds CJ, Watson D. ABC of intensive care: circulatory support. *BMJ* 1999; 318: 1749–1752.

3.8 Ventilatory support

Aim

To partially or completely assist with the work of breathing.
The techniques can be considered under three major headings:

1 Oxygen therapy.
2 Non-invasive positive pressure ventilation (NIPPV).
3 Invasive ventilation.

OXYGEN THERAPY

Mild hypoxaemia

Nasal prongs at 2–3 L/min or a simple mask at 4 L/min.

Moderate to severe hypoxaemia (PaO_2 6.7–8.0 kPa) without CO_2 retention

Simple mask with 4–15 L/min depending on ABGs.

Moderate hypoxaemia with CO_2 retention

Controlled O_2 using a Venturi mask. Start at 24% O_2 and reassess ABGs at 20 min. If PaO_2 <10 kPa and if $PaCO_2$ has risen less than 1.3 kPa, increase to 28%. Recheck ABGs. If hypoxaemia persists, increase the inspired O_2 concentration FiO_2 again and recheck ABGs.

Severe hypoxaemia (PaO_2 <6.7 kPa)

High-flow O_2 via reservoir mask. Get immediate help.

Oxygen therapy

Hypoxia kills quicker than hypercarbia.
All severely ill patients should receive high-flow O_2.
Severely ill patients with chronic obstructive pulmonary disease (COPD) who rely on hypoxic drive to stimulate respiration may benefit from high-flow O_2 initially, buying time to institute other therapy. If they improve, the inspired O_2 concentration should be reduced gradually whilst monitoring ABGs. If the patient does not improve, consideration should be given to assisted ventilation.

NON-INVASIVE POSITIVE PRESSURE VENTILATION

NIPPV is used when increases in inspired O_2 concentration alone fail to maintain adequate PaO_2. Continuous positive airways pressure (CPAP) can be used to recruit collapsed alveoli and increase functional residual capacity, improving lung compliance and reducing the work of breathing.

When the patient makes a respiratory effort, the machine generates positive pressure to assist inspiration.

Indications

NIPPV can be used:
• for patients with acute or acute on chronic hypoxaemia who are not exhausted or in ventilatory failure
• in conditions where alveoli are readily recruited, e.g. acute pulmonary oedema or postoperative atelectasis
• in immunocompromised patients with pneumonia
• in sleep apnoea
• for exacerbations of COPD.

Contraindications

These include:
• Haemodynamic instability or life-threatening dysrhythmias.
• Life-threatening hypoxaemia.
• Exhaustion, impaired mental state or inability to tolerate the mask.

Practical details

NIPPV is applied via a tight-fitting nose or face mask. The usual range of pressure is 2.5–10 cm H_2O. Monitor patient comfort, respiratory rate and ABGs.

Complications

These include:
• Intolerance of face mask, air leaks and ventilator–patient asynchronicity.
• Gastric distension, vomiting and aspiration.
• Eye irritation; conjunctivitis.
• Facial-skin necrosis.

INVASIVE VENTILATION

Invasive ventilation is applied via a tracheal tube or tracheostomy. Ventilation is adjusted by altering minute volume (respiratory rate × tidal volume). Oxygenation is adjusted by altering inspired O_2 concentration and positive end-expiratory pressure (PEEP). This acts in a similar manner to CPAP by recruiting collapsed alveoli and reducing the work of breathing.

Indications

Indications include:
• Airway protection—facial trauma or burns, the unconscious patient.
• Reversible respiratory failure.

• Prophylactic ventilation—after major surgery where some degree of respiratory failure might be expected.
• To avoid or control hypercapnia, e.g. in acute head injury, hepatic coma.
• In 'flail' chest to act as an internal splint.
• To allow removal of secretions, e.g. in Guillain–Barré syndrome, myasthenia gravis.

Practical details

Arrange the settings on the ventilator as follows:
• Tidal volume 10–15 mL/kg in adults.
• Respiratory rate 10–12/min.
• Ratio of inspiratory to expiratory time (I : E ratio) less than 1. For patients with chronic obstructive airway disease (COAD) or asthma, the I : E ratio often needs to be smaller (e.g. 1 : 3) to prevent gas trapping and hyperinflation.

Types of ventilator

Pressure generators

These produce a preset airway pressure or cycle from inspiration to expiration when a preset pressure is reached. If lung compliance falls or airways resistance increases, the tidal volume delivered will fall.

Volume generators

These deliver a fixed tidal volume regardless of changes in lung mechanics. If the lungs become stiffer, the inflation pressure will increase to deliver the same tidal volume.

Cycling

The change from inspiration to expiration is usually time cycled but from expiration to inspiration is either time cycled or may be triggered by the patient if they are breathing spontaneously.

General management

Sedation

It is essential that the patient's breathing is synchronized to that of the ventilator. Failure to do so increases O_2 requirement, increases CO_2 production, reduces cardiac output and is distressing to the patient. Parenteral infusion of narcotics and short-acting benzodiazepines are generally used.

Inhaled gases

Inhaled gases should be warmed, humidified and filtered.

Secretions

Secretions should be cleared by regular physiotherapy and endotracheal suction.

Monitoring

Pulse oximetry and measurement of end-tidal CO_2 provides continuous assessment of oxygenation and ventilation. ABGs should be checked regularly.

Choice of intubation method

Nasotracheal or endotracheal intubation?

The advantages of nasotracheal intubation are:
• It is better tolerated by conscious patients.
• The fixation is more secure.
The disadvantages are:
• Damage to nasal mucosa, alar cartilages and nasal septum.
• Bronchial suction is more difficult.
• Increased resistance to gas flow.
• Increased incidence of sinus infection.

Tracheostomy

Indications include:
• Prolonged ventilation (>2 weeks).
• Expected prolonged absence of protective laryngeal reflexes.
• Retention of secretions.
• Head and neck injuries/surgery.
• Upper airway obstruction.
Tracheostomy has the advantage over intubation of being better tolerated by patients, sedation can be reduced and weaning is often facilitated.
Complications include:
• Displacement of the tube, bleeding and infection.
• Tracheal stenosis.
• Failure of the tracheostomy track to heal.

Complications

Complications include:
• Ventilator-associated pneumonia; ventilated patients have a 10–20 times increased risk of acquiring pneumonia compared with non-ventilated patients.
• Lung damage; overdistension of alveoli and other mechanical effects may exacerbate lung injury. High inflation pressures can cause pneumothorax or subcutaneous emphysema.
• Raised intrathoracic pressure reduces venous return and increases pulmonary vascular resistance. Cardiac output and arterial blood pressure are reduced, heart rate and systemic vascular resistance rise.

• The inherent risks of anaesthesia, sedation and paralysis.

See *Respiratory medicine*, Sections 2.3.2 and 2.3.3.
Hamilton-Farrell MR, Hanson GC. General care of the ventilated patient in the intensive care unit. *Thorax* 1990; 45: 962–969.
Hillberg RE, Johnson DC. Noninvasive ventilation. *N Engl J Med* 1997; 24: 1746–1752.
Ponte J. Indications for mechanical ventilation. *Thorax* 1990; 45: 885–890.

3.9 Airway management

Aim

To recognize and treat airway compromise.

Indications

Recognition of airway compromise depends on the following basic and life-saving techniques:
Look, listen and feel.
• Look for chest movement.
• Listen and feel for air movement at the nose and mouth.
• Stridor, gurgling and snoring all suggest an airway at risk. All unconscious patients are at risk:

• A patient with a GCS of <8 will need endotracheal intubation unless a cause can be rapidly found and corrected.
• Patients with a GCS of 8–12 may need basic adjuncts to maintain airway patency.

Airway compromise results in rapid hypoxia and secondary brain injury. Airway management is the first priority in basic life support (airway, breathing, circulation). However, be wary of patients who are spontaneously ventilating but who cannot protect their airway because of a reduction in conscious level.

Practical details

Opening the airway

Head tilt/chin lift

1 Loss of muscle control leads to occlusion of the airway by the tongue, epiglottis and soft palate.
2 With the patient supine, extend the head on the neck by placing one hand on the forehead and pushing backwards.
3 Place the fingers of the other hand under the tip of the jaw and lift the chin upwards (Fig. 55a).

Jaw thrust

1 Place the fingers of both hands behind the angles of the mandible. Use upward pressure to lift the jaw forward (Fig. 55b).

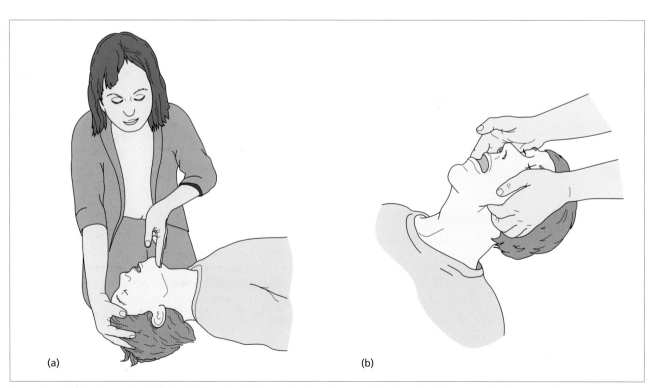

(a)
(b)

Fig. 55 Opening the airway. (a) Head tilt/chin lift method. Place one hand on the patient's forehead and the other under the point of the patient's chin. Tilt the head back to open the airway. (b) Jaw thrust method. With the index and middle fingers behind the angle of the mandible, apply upward and forward pressure to lift the jaw.

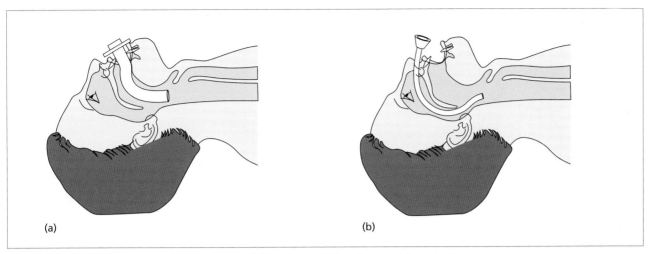

Fig. 56 Basic adjuncts to airway control. (a) Oropharyngeal airway *in situ*. (b) Nasopharyngeal airway *in situ*.

2 This is the preferred technique when cervical spine injury is suspected.

> In patients who have a suspected neck injury, the jaw thrust method is preferred as it results in less neck movement, but remember, death is more commonly caused by airway obstruction in such patients than from damage due to neck movement.

Removing obstructions from the oropharynx

1 Solid foreign material should be removed using Magill forceps or a finger sweep under direct vision.
2 Semisolid material or liquid should be removed using a Yankauer sucker.

Basic adjuncts to airway control

Oropharyngeal and nasopharyngeal airways help to prevent occlusion of the pharynx by the tongue and soft tissues (Fig. 56). Patients with preserved laryngeal reflexes will generally not tolerate an oropharyngeal airway but may tolerate a nasopharyngeal one.

Insertion of an oropharyngeal airway

1 Select an airway that corresponds in length to the distance between the corner of the patient's mouth and the angle of the jaw.
2 Open the patient's mouth.
3 Introduce the airway upside down and rotate it 180° as it passes into the oropharynx.
4 Reassess the airway.

> Be aware of potential problems with oropharyngeal airways:
> • Incorrect insertion of the airway can exacerbate the problem by pushing the tongue further back.
> • In the presence of laryngeal reflexes, insertion of an oropharyngeal airway can trigger vomiting and laryngospasm.

Insertion of a nasopharyngeal airway

1 Select an airway with an external diameter similar to the patient's little finger.
2 Place a safety pin through the external flange of the airway to prevent it being inhaled. Lubricate the airway.
3 Check patency of the nostrils and for the presence of septal deviation. Use the nostril that seems easiest!
4 Insert the airway perpendicularly to the nostril, along the floor of the nose.
5 The airway should pass easily such that the flange comes to rest at the nostril. If it does not, remove it and try the other nostril.
6 Reassess the airway.

> **Nasopharyngeal airways**
> Do not insert a nasopharyngeal airway if there is a suspected fracture of the base of the skull.

> Remember that O_2 is free and should be given to all patients with decreased conscious levels unless specifically contraindicated.

> **Ventilatory support**
> Ventilatory support must be provided if the patient has inadequate or absent ventilation. In the short term, this can be provided by mouth-to-mouth, mouth-to-mask or bag–valve–mask ventilation (the latter is a two-person technique unless you are experienced). It is more important to ventilate the patient than for the inexperienced to attempt intubation. Get help!

> The 1998 European Resuscitation Council guidelines for adult single rescuer basic life support. A statement from the Working Group on Basic Life Support. *Resuscitation* 1998; 37: 67–80.

4 Self-assessment

Answers on pp. 115–19.

Question 1

A 48-year-old man with no significant past medical history and on no regular medication presents with central chest pain that radiates to his neck. For 48 hrs prior to admission he has felt feverish, with headache and generalized aches in his muscles and joints. He has smoked 20 cigarettes a day for about 30 years. His father died at the age of 74 years following a heart attack. He does not look unwell, but is febrile (37.8 degrees). Examination is otherwise unremarkable. His ECG is shown (see Fig. 57). The most likely diagnosis is:

A acute inferior myocardial infarction
B acute inferior myocardial infarction with lateral extension
C pericarditis
D pulmonary embolism
E myocarditis

Question 2

A 68-year-old man presents with one hour of central chest pain. His ECG is shown (see Fig. 58). The diagnosis is:

A pericarditis
B acute inferior myocardial infarction with posterior extension
C acute anterior myocardial infarction with lateral extension
D acute anterior myocardial infarction
E acute inferior myocardial infarction

Question 3

A 70-year-old man presents with a history of feeling faint on several occasions in the last month, although he has never collapsed. On examination his pulse is 40/min. His ECG is shown (see Fig. 59). The diagnosis is:

A sinus bradycardia
B sick sinus syndrome
C 1st degree AV block
D 2nd degree AV block
E 3rd degree AV block

Question 4

A 48-year-old man presents with 48 hours of fever, rigors, breathlessness and bilateral pleuritic chest pain which came on as he thought that he was recovering from an

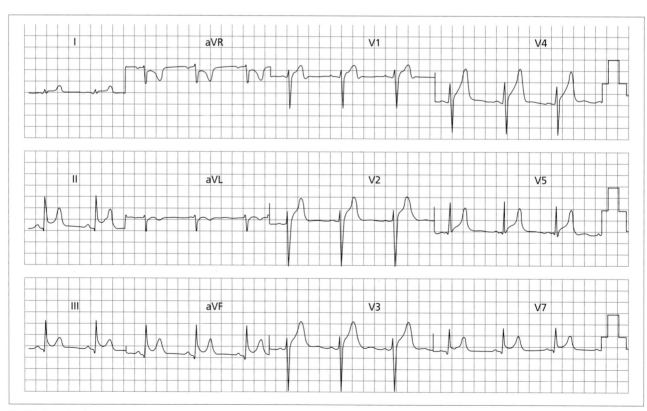

Fig. 57 Question 1.

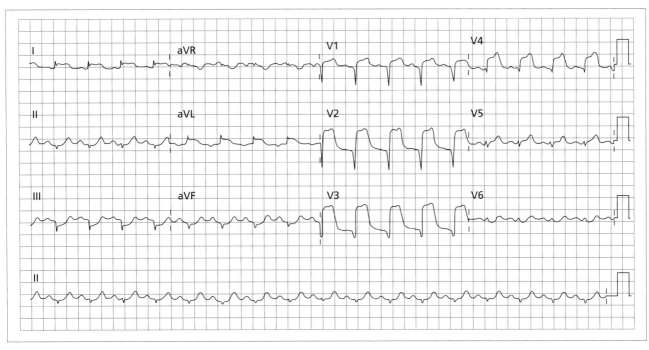

Fig. 58 Question 2.

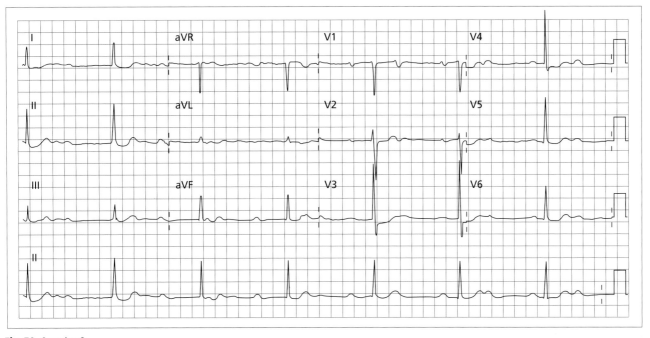

Fig. 59 Question 3.

attack of 'flu. He is very unwell, with cyanosis, pulse 120/min, respiratory rate 24/min and BP 100/60 mmHg. His chest radiograph is shown (see Fig. 60). The diagnosis is:

A lobar pneumonia (right upper lobe)

B lobar pneumonia (right middle lobe)

C lobar pneumonia (right upper lobe) with left pneumothorax

D lobar pneumonia (right middle lobe) with left pneumothorax

E lobar pneumonia (right middle lobe) with loculated right pleural effusion

Question 5

You are walking onto a ward when you notice that a 78-year-old man has collapsed in his bed. Your first two actions should be:

A call the cardiac arrest team

B defibrillate (200 J)

C check that the situation is safe

D check responsiveness (shake and shout)

E check breathing (observe for movement of the chest)

F open airway (head tilt/chin lift)

G start chest compression

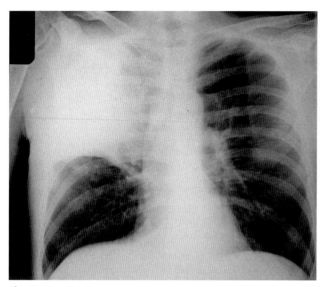

Fig. 60 Question 4.

H check for pulse (carotid)
I give precordial thump
J check for pulse (femoral)

Question 6

A 48-year-old man presents with 40 minutes of cardiac chest pain. Which two of the following ECG criteria are indications for thrombolysis?

A 2 mm or more elevation of the ST segment in any one standard ECG lead
B atrial fibrillation
C 2 mm or more ST segment depression in two or more standard ECG leads
D 2 mm or more elevation of ST segments in two or more contiguous praecordial leads
E new right bundle branch block
F ventricular tachycardia
G 1 mm or more elevation of ST segments in two or more standard ECG leads
H 2 mm or more elevation of ST segments in any two ECG leads
I 1 mm or more elevation of ST segments in any two ECG leads
J 1 mm or more elevation of ST segments in two or more contiguous praecordial leads

Question 7

A 22-year-old man presents to the Accident and Emergency department claiming to have taken a large quantity of paracetamol 24 hours previously. He washed the tablets down with vodka. Which two of the following statements are correct?
A measuring paracetamol levels at 24 hours is of no use
B *N*-acetyl cysteine should be witheld until plasma paracetamol levels are known.

C the prognostic accuracy of the treatment nomogram is less certain at 24 hours post-ingestion.
D methionine can be given if the patient is intolerant of *N*-acetyl cysteine (NAC).
E clinical symptoms may occur > 24 hours post-ingestion.
F if the urea and electrolytes are normal, the patient can be sent home.
G even at 24 hours, activated charcoal should be given as gastric transit time is prolonged by paracetamol.
H the measurement of alanine transferase is of prognostic value.
I if he drank more than two units of alcohol with the overdose, he is at greater risk.
J if he is obese, he is at greater risk from the effects of the overdose

Question 8

A 40-year-woman presents after a deliberate overdose of paracetamol. Which two of the following are suggestive of the development of acute liver failure 48 hours after a paracetamol overdose?
A prothrombin time > 60 seconds, control 12 seconds
B albumin > 30 g/ litre
C alanine aminotransferase (ALT) ten times upper limit of laboratory normal range
D evidence of metabolic acidosis
E hyperglycaemia
F hypokalaemia
G elevated C-reactive protein (CRP)
H leucocytosis
I erythrocyte sedimentation rate (ESR) > 50 mm/hr
J thrombocytosis

Question 9

A 22-year-old woman with known severe asthma presents to the emergency department complaining of acute breathlessness for the last 4 hours. She has had no response from her ordinary medication and is getting distressed. The ambulance crew have given 100% oxygen and a salbutamol nebuliser. Which two of the following statements concerning the management of acute severe asthma are correct?
A aminophylline improves the ventilation/perfusion mismatch.
B hyperkalaemia commonly follows treatment with beta-2 agonists
C patients require high right ventricular filling pressures.
D 28–35% oxygen should be used for patients with hypercapnia to avoid progressive hypoventilation.
E intravenous beta-2 agonists are contraindicated as they exacerbate tachycardia
F the most important investigation is the peak expiratory flow rate
G a normal arterial carbon dioxide concentration suggests the alternative diagnosis of hysterical hyperventilation

H low dose diazepam is useful for alleviating anxiety

I the degree of pulsus paradoxus correlates with the severity of the attack

J absence of wheeze excludes the diagnosis

Question 10

A 72-year-old woman has been admitted to the ward via the Emergency Department. She was found collapsed at home, semiconscious. Her Glasgow coma score (GCS) is currently 10 and she is receiving oxygen via a venturi mask. You notice that she has stridor with marked inspiratory effort. Which two of the following statements regarding basic airway management are correct?

A the length of an oropharyngeal airway should correspond to the length of the patient's little finger

B oropharyngeal airways are contraindicated in patients with a base of skull fracture

C patients with preserved laryngeal reflexes will not tolerate a nasopharyngeal tube

D insertion of an oropharyngeal airway can trigger laryngospasm

E a nasopharyngeal airway cannot be used if the nose is fractured

F both nasopharyngeal and oropharyngeal airways can provide a definitive airway for comatose patients

G nasopharyngeal and oropharyngeal airways should be used when a jaw thrust is contraindicated

H the diameter of a nasopharyngeal tube should be similar to the diameter of the patient's little finger

I a head-tilt chin lift produces less neck movement than a jaw thrust manoeuvre

J vomitus should be removed from the airway using a blind finger-sweep

Question 11

Non-invasive methods of ventilation (NIV) are increasingly used for patients with a variety of acute and chronic medical conditions. A 75-year-old smoker with end-stage chronic obstructive pulmonary disease is admitted. He has been using NIV at home. Which two of the following statements regarding non-invasive ventilation are correct?

A It is not indicated for patients with terminal conditions.

B It should only be used with a nasogastric tube in situ.

C It reduces expiratory effort.

D It can cause facial skin necrosis.

E It can be used for comatose patients.

F It may be of benefit for patients with sleep apnoea.

G It increases the work of breathing.

H It should only be used if the patient has a definitive airway

I It can be used only for type 1 respiratory failure

J It reduces functional residual capacity

Question 12

A 67-year-old man is on coronary care following an inferior myocardial infarct. He has had a temporary transvenous pacemaker inserted for Mobitz type II heart block. He suddenly becomes light-headed with chest pain. The cardiac monitor shows complete heart block with a rate of 20 bpm. What should be your first two actions?

A call the cardiac arrest team

B ask him to cough repeatedly

C give a precordial thump

D check the lead connections on the pacemaker

E institute external pacing

F obtain a 12 lead electrocardiogram

G increase the pacemaker voltage to maximum

H start an isoprenaline infusion

I give streptokinase 1.5 MU intravenously

J give morphine 5–10 mg intravenously

Question 13

A 40-year-old woman presents four hours after an overdose of amitriptyline and diazepam. On examination her Glasgow Coma Scale score is 10. She has dilated pupils, a blood pressure of 100/70 mmHg and a pulse of 140 beats per minute. Her SaO_2 (pulse oximetry) is 95% and her blood glucose (finger prick test) is 7.0 mmol/l. Which is the most appropriate other immediate investigation?

A CT brain scan

B serum urea and electrolytes

C ECG

D serum paracetamol level

E serum salicylate level

Question 14

A 35-year-old woman presents 2 hours after collapsing at home with severe headache. On examination she is drowsy and has neck stiffness. Her temperature is 37.5°C. She has a mild right hemiparesis. Which of the following is the most appropriate first diagnostic investigation?

A CT brain scan

B lumbar puncture and examination of the cerebrospinal fluid

C four-vessel angiography

D MR angiogram

E MR brain scan

Question 15

A 50-year-old man presents with lethargy and palpitations. His ECG shows tented T waves, small/absent P waves, and broad QRS complexes. Investigations reveal:

Serum sodium	144 mmol/L (Normal range: 137–144)

Serum potassium	7.9 mmol/L (3.5–4.9)
Serum bicarbonate	9 mmol/L (20–28)
Serum urea	40.5 mmol/L (2.5–7.5)
Serum creatinine	510 μmol/L (60–110)

The best immediate therapy is:

A intravenous calcium gluconate

B intravenous dextrose and insulin

C intravenous sodium bicarbonate

D nebulised salbutamol

E rectal calcium resonium

Question 16

A 75-year-old man is admitted to hospital. He is receiving warfarin as prophylaxis following a DVT. His international normalised ratio (INR) has been stable at 2–2.5 for the past 8 weeks. While in hospital his INR increases to >8: which of the following drugs prescribed in hospital could cause his increased INR?

A ciprofloxacin

B aspirin

C carbamazepine

D rifampicin

E co-dydramol

Question 17

A 50-year-old woman presents to the emergency department with a short history of severe occipital headache, vomiting and impaired balance. Her past medical history includes hypertension. On examination she has nystagmus to the right, ataxia of her right limbs and gait ataxia. What is the most likely diagnosis?

A basal ganglia haemorrhage

B subdural haemorrhage

C left temporal lobe haemorrhage

D pontine haemorrhage

E cerebellar haemorrhage

Question 18

A 48-year-old man is admitted to hospital with an anterior myocardial infarct. He receives treatment with thrombolysis, aspirin, a beta blocker and a statin. He makes good progress and is about to be discharged on day 7 when he develops chest pain. This is different in nature from the pain that precipitated his admission. You cannot decide clinically whether it is ischaemic cardiac pain. In deciding how to investigate, which one of the following statements regarding troponins is correct?

A elevated plasma concentrations are specific markers for ischaemic heart disease

B elevated plasma concentrations would typically be found two weeks after an acute myocardial infarction.

C the sensitivity of troponins for cardiac muscle damage is similar to that of CK-MB.

D reduced plasma concentrations are typically found in patients who are in atrial fibrillation.

E troponins have a key role in the decision regarding thrombolysis in patients presenting with chest pain.

Question 19

A 33-year-old woman presents with sudden onset pleuritic chest pain that came on while she was lifting her 18-month-old son. She complains of feeling short of breath. She is otherwise fit and well, is on no medication, but smokes 10 cigarettes per day. Clinical examination is normal, as are chest x-ray and resting ECG. Pulse oximetry reveals that her oxygen saturation breathing room air is 97%. A Vidas D-dimer is less than 500 ng/ml, i.e. within the normal range. The most likely diagnosis is:

A musculoskeletal chest pain

B pericarditis

C pulmonary embolism

D atypical pneumonia

E unstable angina

Question 20

A 55-year-old man with a history of severe asthma and ischaemic heart disease is brought to the Emergency Department complaining of palpitations and syncope. On examination he has a weak, regular pulse with a rate of 180 / minute with a blood pressure of 110/70 mmHg. A 12 lead ECG reveals a broad complex tachycardia. Which of the following statements is correct?

A absence of capture or fusion beats on a long rhythm strip is strongly suggestive of supraventricular tachycardia (SVT) with aberrant conduction

B SVT is more likely than ventricular tachycardia (VT) if the patient gives a history of recent myocardial infarction

C intravenous adenosine should be used to distinguish SVT from VT

D QRS calibre greater than 0.2s is usually indicative of VT

E SVT with aberrant conduction is unlikely if a recent ECG showed no evidence of bundle branch block

Question 21

A 45-year-old man with chronic alcoholic liver disease was admitted earlier in the day following a large haematemesis. He was treated with intravenous terlipressin and urgent endoscopy was arranged after initial fluid resuscitation and correction of a mild coagulopathy with fresh frozen plasma. Endoscopy revealed bleeding oesophageal varices, which were injected with sclerosant with apparently good effect. He has been stable on the ward for the past 6 hours, but you are called to see him in the early hours of the following morning because he has had a further 500 ml haematemesis, and his blood pressure has dropped from 130/90 mmHg to 90/50 mmHg. Which of the following measures would be most appropriate in addition to fluid resuscitation?

A urgent repeat endoscopy and sclerotherapy

B change terlipressin to octreotide

C administer 10 mg vitamin K intravenously

D insert Sengstaken tube, inflate gastric balloon and apply traction

E urgent surgical intervention

Question 22

A 45-year-old man with a history of alcohol-related chronic liver disease presents following a 400 ml fresh haematemesis. On examination he is jaundiced with palmar erythema and marked ascites. Pulse is 120 beats per minute and blood pressure 100/70 mmHg. In addition to fluid resuscitation, which of the following treatments is most likely to be beneficial in his initial management, while awaiting upper GI endoscopy?

A ranitidine 50 mg intravenously

B omeprazole 40 mg intravenous bolus

C tranexamic acid 1 g intravenously

D terlipressin 2 mg intravenous bolus

E propranolol 40 mg orally

Question 23

A 26-year-old woman presents with a week's history of progressive numbness and weakness in her lower limbs. Which of the following suggests a diagnosis of Guillain-Barré syndrome (GBS)?

A optic atrophy on fundoscopy

B a sensory level

C ankle weakness with saddle area sensory loss

D autonomic dysfunction

E proximal weakness > distal

Question 24

A frail 73-year-old woman is admitted via the Accident and Emergency department with agitation, restlessness and confusion. On examination she is apyrexial and has no chest signs. Abdominal examination is normal and rectal examination reveals a small amount of normal stool. Her son reports that she had been staying with him for a long weekend just to give her a break, but unfortunately she had forgotten to bring her medications with her. He says that she has a long history of agitation and anxiety. Her blood tests are all normal. Urine dipstick testing for nitrites and leucocytes is negative. The most likely cause for her confused state is:

A urinary tract infection

B chest infection

C alcohol withdrawal

D constipation

E benzodiazepine withdrawal

Question 25

A 47-year-old woman with a past history of relapsing-remitting multiple sclerosis presents to the acute medical take following a flare-up of her condition. Which of the following statements regarding steroid treatment is NOT true?

A corticosteroid treatment may limit the duration of visual loss due to optic neuritis

B avascular necrosis of the femoral head is a recognised complication of corticosteroid treatment

C corticosteroid treatment may reduce the frequency of future relapses

D oral corticosteroid treatment has no impact on rate of recovery from a relapse

E 1 g methylprednisolone daily for 3 days is an appropriate dose

Question 26

An elderly man is brought into the Accident and Emergency department by ambulance because he had been found wandering down his street early in the morning. He gives a fluent history of his past life, but is unable to explain what he had been doing. On examination he smells of alcohol. He has nystagmus and bilateral lateral gaze palsies. Which of the following statements is NOT correct?

A the lesions are in the mamillary bodies and thalamus

B his red cell transketolase is low

C examination of his pupils is normal

D all of his deficits will resolve with 3 days of parenteral thiamine

E a CT scan of his head is likely to be normal

Question 27

A 25-year-old woman presents to the Accident and Emergency department 1 hour after consuming 28 × 500 mg paracetamol tablets. Which of the following statements is true?

A if the INR is normal on a sample taken four hours from the time of ingestion, liver damage is unlikely to occur

B alcohol ingestion at the time of consumption of paracetamol is an indication for N-acetyl-cysteine treatment if paracetamol level at 4 hours exceeds the 'high-risk' line

C activated charcoal may be beneficial if given immediately

D onset of tinnitus may be an early symptom of liver failure

E deterioration in conscious level within the first 24 hours usually suggests hepatic encephalopathy

Question 28

A 50-year-old man presents with sudden onset shortness of breath and pleuritic chest pain. He has a CT pulmonary angiogram, which shows a large pulmonary embolus.

Which of the following is NOT an indication for thrombolysis in this patient?

A cardiac arrest

B falling blood pressure

C D-dimer greater than 4000

D engorgement of neck veins

E right ventricular gallop

Question 29

A 28-year-old woman with type I diabetes mellitus develops abdominal pain and vomiting after eating a stale chicken sandwich. She presents to hospital two days later. Which of the following statements concerning diabetic ketoacidosis is NOT correct?

A it may present as an acute abdomen

B serum amylase may be elevated without evidence of pancreatitis

C the white cell count may be elevated without evidence of infection.

D the anion gap is normal.

E although serum potassium is often raised, total body potassium is reduced.

Question 30

An 18-year-old woman is admitted having deliberately taken a large overdose of her father's atenolol tablets. Which of the following statements is NOT true?

A dizziness is a common feature of beta-blocker overdose

B a temporary pacing wire may be required.

C atropine should not be given due to the risk of causing tachycardia

D glucagon is a useful therapy in the management of beta-blocker overdose

E paracetamol levels should be measured

Question 31

An 18-year-old woman is brought to the Accident and Emergency department by a friend, who says that she has been ill for 24 hours with 'flu-like symptoms and headache. She is unwell, drowsy and has a purpuric rash on her arms. Your immediate action is to:

A order a CT scan of her brain

B perform a lumbar puncture

C take blood cultures and await result

D give aciclovir 10 mg/kg intravenously

E give cefotaxime 2 g intravenously

Question 32

A 27-year-old woman develops difficulty breathing and her lips and tongue swell about five minutes after starting to eat a curry. She is brought to the Accident and Emergency department by ambulance. She is cyanosed and wheezing. Aside from high flow oxygen via a reservoir bag, which of the following treatments would be your top priority?

A hydrocortisone 200 mg intravenously

B chlorpheniramine 10 mg intravenously

C epinephrine (adrenaline)—0.5 ml of 1/1000 solution intravenously

D epinephrine (adrenaline)—0.5 ml of 1/1000 solution intramuscularly

E salbutamol 5 mg nebulized

Question 33

An 82-year-old man is admitted after a syncopal episode. His pulse rate is 40/min and ECG confirms complete (3rd degree) heart block. His pulse slows to 24/min and he feels very faint. Whilst arrangements are being made for temporary pacing you give:

A adrenaline 0.5 mg intravenous bolus

B isoprenaline 50 mg intravenous bolus

C atropine 0.5 mg intravenous bolus

D atropine 5 mg intravenous bolus

E isoprenaline 500 mg intravenous bolus

Question 34

A man is brought to the Accident and Emergency department by ambulance. He is unconscious (GCS 5) with pin-point pupils and a slow respiratory rate. Immediate specific treatment should be:

A naloxone (0.4 mg) intravenously, repeated if no effect

B N-acetyl cysteine (150 mg/kg over 15 min) intravenously, then 50 mg/kg over 4 hours, then 100 mg/kg over 16 hours

C dextrose (50 ml of 50% solution) intravenously, repeated if no effect

D naloxone (4 mg) intravenously, repeated if no effect

E insert stomach tube (after securing airway) and give activated charcoal

Question 35

A 38-year-old man presents with acute renal failure and serum creatinine 988 μmol/l. A house physician performs arterial blood gas analysis (breathing air) and finds pH 7.12, pO_2 12.8 kPa, pCO_2 3.2 kPa, BE –12 mmol/l. He asks you what a base excess of –12 means. You reply:

A it means that the serum bicarbonate concentration is 12 mmol/l

B it means that the serum bicarbonate concentration is 12 mmol/l below normal

C it means that the pH is 0.12 units below the lower limit of the normal range for the machine being used

D an algorithm is used to predict what pH would arise in normal blood in the presence of the pCO_2 actually measured, the base excess being the amount of acid that would have to be added or removed to obtain the pH actually measured

E an algorithm is used to predict what pH would arise in normal blood in the presence of the pCO_2 actually measured, the base excess being the amount of base that would have to be added or removed to obtain the pH actually measured

Question 36
A 38-year-old asthmatic woman presents with an acute attack. Her arterial blood gases breathing air are as follows: pH 7.36, pO_2 9.8 kPa, pCO_2 5.2 kPa. These are most likely to mean:
A the attack is not severe
B she should be given supplemental oxygen, but is unlikely to need a high FiO_2 to achieve normoxia
C cardiorespiratory arrest could be imminent
D her respiratory effort may be failing because she is getting tired
E she could have had a pneumothorax

Question 37
A 28-year-old man with asthma presents with an acute attack. He is very breathless and cannot complete sentences. Which of the following is the best immediate management?
A nebulised salbutamol (5 mg) driven with air
B organise chest radiograph to exclude pneumothorax
C nebulised salbutamol (5 mg) driven with high flow oxygen via reservoir bag
D nebulised salbutamol (50 mg) driven with 35% oxygen
E nebulised salbutamol (5 mg) driven with 35% oxygen

Question 38
A 72-year-old man is admitted to the coronary care unit with an acute myocardial infarction. He suffers a cardiac arrest. Basic life support is being given as you arrive. The ECG monitor reveals ventricular fibrillation (VF). The first defibrillation attempt should be made at:

A 200 J
B 400 J
C 360 J
D 20 J
E 100 J

Question 39
A 35-year-old woman presents 6 hours after a deliberate overdose of paracetamol. The paracetamol level at 6 hours is above the treatment line. Thirty minutes after starting an infusion of *N*-acetyl cysteine (NAC) she becomes flushed and hypotensive with a blood pressure of 80/55 mmHg. The infusion is stopped immediately and 500 ml IV 0.9% saline administered over 30 minutes. Which of the following is the correct ongoing management?
A IV chlorpheniramine and restart NAC infusion at lowest rate once symptoms resolved
B IV chlorpromazine and restart NAC infusion at lowest rate once symptoms resolved
C IV chlorpheniramine and give 2.5 g of oral methionine
D IV chlorpromazine and give 2.5 g of oral methionine
E withhold treatment and recheck paracetamol level at 12 hours

Question 40
A 21-year-old man reports having taken an overdose of 'some tablets'. For which of the following would you NOT use activated charcoal within the first hour?
A paracetamol
B aspirin
C diazepam
D atenolol
E lithium

Answers to Self-assessment

Answer to Question 1

C

In the context of this clinical history, which clearly suggests a viral illness, the widespread changes to ST-segments and T-waves suggest pericarditis.

With a different history the possibility of acute inferior myocardial infarction with lateral extension would require consideration.

Answer to Question 2

C

The appearances are typical of acute anterior myocardial infarction, with gross ST-segment elevation and early Q wave formation in leads V1-4.

Answer to Question 3

E

The ECG shows 3rd degree (complete) heart block, with P waves completely dissociated from the QRS complexes. The narrow QRS complexes indicate that the focus for ventricular activity is high in the ventricular conduction system.

Answer to Question 4

A

There is dense consolidation of the right upper lobe, caused in this case by staphylococcal pneumonia following the 'flu.

Answer to Question 5

C, D

Adult basic life support involves:
(1) Check that the situation is safe.
(2) Check responsiveness: shake and shout.
(3) Open airway: head tilt / chin lift.
(4) Check breathing: look / listen.
(5) If breathing: recovery position.
(6) If not breathing: assess circulation: 10 seconds only.
(7) Circulation present: continue rescue breathing.
(8) Circulation not present: compress chest: 100 / min, 15:2 ratio.

Answer to Question 6

D, G

The other recognised ECG criterion for thrombolysis is new left bundle branch block.

Answer to Question 7

C, E

Levels should always be measured in cases of paracetamol overdose, but if a clinically significant quantity of paracetamol seems to have been taken, start *N*-acetyl cysteine (NAC) whilst waiting for the results—it can be stopped if it proves to be inappropriate. Clotting, liver function, renal function and electrolytes should all be checked: the best prognostic indicator is the INR.

Intolerance to NAC is rare: most reactions to it are mild and can be overcome by slowing the rate of infusion. For patients who are truly intolerant, methionine can be given up to 12 hours after paracetamol ingestion.

Patients who are anorexic for any reason, who drink significantly (>21 units/wk for men, >14 units/wk for women) or who are on enzyme-inducing drugs are at greater risk from paracetamol overdose.

Answer to Question 8

A, D

A prolonged prothrombin time is a poor prognostic factor: there is a definite risk of acute liver failure and a need for expert toxicological and hepatological advice. Metabolic acidosis, which can be detected by arterial blood gas analysis, rising venous lactate or falling venous bicarbonate, also indicate deteriorating liver function and the need for specialist advice/transfer.

Answer to Question 9

C, I

Aminophylline is a pulmonary vasodilator and can worsen VQ mismatch. Beta-2 agonists are a recognised treatment for hyperkalaemia as they drive potassium into the cells. Patients with acute asthma are usually dry: because of high intrathoracic pressure they need a high right ventricular filling pressure to maintain cardiac output. Never use low flow oxygen in this context: hypoxia kills, hypercarbia merely intoxicates. If an acute asthmatic is hypercarbic they need ventilation. IV beta-2 agonists can be life saving in patients who are too breathless to be helped by nebulisers.

The most important investigation is arterial blood gas analysis as this will give information on carbon dioxide concentration and pH. A normal carbon dioxide level is a worrying sign—it suggests a tiring asthmatic. Hyperventilation should lower the carbon dioxide concentration.

Low dose diazepam is likely to result in your appearance in a coroner's court—sedation is contraindicated, unless the patient is mechanically ventilated. The degree of pulsus paradoxus (fall in systolic blood pressure during inspiration) does correlate with the severity of attack, but use the arterial blood gases as a guide to therapy and not repeated measurement of paradox.

Answer to Question 10

D, H

The first step in basic airway management is to open the airway. This should be done with a head-tilt chin lift, unless there is suggestion of a neck injury when a jaw-thrust manoeuvre is preferred. Material in the oropharynx should be removed under direct vision. Oropharyngeal (OPA) and nasopharyngeal (NPA) airways are useful adjuncts but do not provide a definitive airway for unconscious patients.

A quick way to size an NPA is to choose one with an external diameter similar to the patient's little finger. NPAs are contraindicated in base of skull fractures. If there is a nasal fracture, the most patent nostril should be chosen. NPAs are generally better tolerated than OPAs and can be used in patients where the laryngeal reflexes are preserved.

OPAs should be sized with the length corresponding to the distance from the angle of the patient's mouth to the angle of the jaw. Inserting OPAs can trigger vomiting and laryngospasm.

Answer to Question 11
D, F
Modern non-invasive ventilation (NIV) can provide support for patients with both type 1 and type 2 respiratory failure and is increasingly being used to support patients with conditions such as motor neurone disease, where it is mainly CO_2 clearance that is the problem. It should not be used for patients with immediate life-threatening hypoxia or ventilatory failure.

NIV should not be used in those who are comatose: it does not provide a definitive airway and the patient would be at risk of aspiration. NIV increases the risk of aspiration because raised inspiratory pressure can result in aerophagia: a nasogastric tube may be beneficial if the patient has problems with gastric distension, but this is not required in most cases.

Patients with sleep apnoea suffer from recurrent episodes of arterial desaturation. The application of continuous positive airway pressure helps to reduce these. Expiratory effort is increased as the patient is expiring against resistance, but inspiratory effort and the overall work of breathing are reduced. Functional residual capacity is increased. Common complications of NIV include claustrophobia, gastric distension and eye irritation. Continual pressure from a tight fitting mask may result in skin necrosis.

Answer to Question 12
D, G
The patient's symptoms result from his bradycardia and the pacemaker is failing to capture. The first thing to do is to check the leads. If they are connected, then the pacemaker voltage should be increased to maximum which may enable it to capture.

The threshold for pacing increases with time and should be checked at least daily. If capture occurs, arrangements should be made to reposition the pacemaker lead. If it does not, external pacing should be instituted. Cough and percussion pacing are emergency measures that occasionally work. Isoprenaline can also be effective.

Answer to Question 13
C
Tricyclic overdose can cause coma, convulsions and arrhythmias in serious cases. The single most important investigation to determine prognosis and guide therapy is a 12 lead ECG: a QRS duration >160 ms is associated with high risk of arrhythmias and the patient should be managed on a CCU / HDU. Always check for other poisons in cases of polypharmacy overdose, also check arterial blood gases for signs of hypoventilation and acidosis, but these are not the most appropriate immediate investigations in this case.

Answer to Question 14
A
The history suggests a subarachnoid haemorrhage (SAH). Urgent CT brain scan will identify more than 95% of patients with suspected subarachnoid haemorrhage if performed within 1–2 days after headache onset. Lumbar puncture is potentially dangerous in a case where there might be raised intracranial pressure and will add no extra information if brain CT shows definite evidence of extravasated blood. If CT is negative and there are no contraindications, then LP should be performed.

When the patient has stabilised, four vessel angiography will be needed to identify the source of the bleeding, which may be amenable to endovascular or surgical treatment. CT imaging is superior to MRI in acute SAH because of the speed of investigation and availability. MRI imaging becomes more useful if presentation is delayed because CT sensitivity for subarachnoid blood rapidly declines after the first few days (>4). MR angiography is without risks and reasonably sensitive (90%): it is useful for screening people at risk of intracranial aneurysms, but less suitable for patients with subarachnoid haemorrhage.

Answer to Question 15
A
The immediate priority is to protect the heart from the effects of hyperkalaemia. This can best be done with intravenous calcium gluconate 10% 10–20 mls IV which acts instantly to 'stabilise' the cardiac membranes. The other options listed are valuable treatments for hyperkalaemia, but are not the best immediate therapy in this context because they all take time to have an effect.

Answer to Question 16
A
The commonly prescribed antibiotics clarithromycin, ciprofloxacin and metronidazole enhance the anticoagulant effect of warfarin, whereas rifampicin (a potent enzyme inducing drug) diminishes the anticoagulant effect.

Although aspirin may increase the likelihood of bleeding due to its antiplatelet and gastric irritant effects, it should not cause prolongation of the INR; other non-steroidal anti-inflammatory (NSAIDs), especially azapropazone, may cause prolongation of the INR.

Carbamazepine, primidone and phenobarbitone induce liver enzymes and therefore reduce anticoagulant effect, while valproate probably increases the INR. The effect of phenytoin is unpredictable, as both prolongation and reduction of the INR have been reported.

Unlike co-proxamol, which causes prolongation of the INR, co-dydramol has no significant effect on warfarin metabolism.

Answer to Question 17
E

She has posterior circulation signs, in particular right cerebellar signs. The immediate priority must be to exclude an acute cerebellar haemorrhage that may need surgical intervention.

Answer to Question 18
B

Troponins I and T may remain elevated for up to 3 weeks after myocardial infarction and hence are not very useful for repeat events during this period, unless a rising plasma concentration can be demonstrated.

Troponins are specific markers for cardiac muscle damage, but not specific markers of ischaemia: other conditions, e.g. myocarditis, may also produce an elevated level. A good history along with ECG changes is the only evidence-based criteria on which to base a decision on thrombolysis. Troponins are more sensitive than CK-MB in the detection of minor degrees of cardiac muscle damage and can be used as prognostic markers in the risk stratification of Acute Coronary Syndromes.

Answer to Question 19
A

The history suggests a mechanical cause and all routine investigations are normal. The negative Vidas D-dimer result makes pulmonary embolism very unlikely in the context of a low probability presentation, i.e. no risk factors and an alternative diagnosis.

Answer to Question 20
D

Although the presence of capture and fusion beats is pathognomonic of VT, they are rarely seen and their absence cannot be relied upon to rule out the diagnosis. Broad complex tachycardia in the first week after a myocardial infarction is proven to be ventricular in origin in over 90% of cases. Adenosine may induce bronchospasm and should be avoided in patients with a history of asthma. The absence of bundle branch block on a recent ECG is an unreliable indicator of the source of the tachycardia, since bundle branch block is frequently rate-related, and often resolves on termination of the dysrhythmia.

Answer to Question 21
D

Balloon tamponade is the most effective treatment for control of variceal bleeding if endoscopic therapy has failed. Even though the varices were bleeding from within the oesophagus, inflation of the gastric balloon with application of traction usually stops the bleeding by compressing the vessels as they cross the gastrooesophageal junction. Rarely, inflation of the oesophageal balloon may be required.

It is unlikely that repeat endoscopy would prevent on-going bleeding if he has already received successful sclerotherapy, unless there was doubt about the source of bleeding previously. Octreotide is less effective than terlipressin in controlling portal pressure, and therefore switching therapy is unlikely to be helpful. Although the effects of the fresh frozen plasma administered earlier will probably have worn off, vitamin K is unlikely to help as the coagulopathy is probably due to synthetic dysfunction rather than vitamin K deficiency. Surgical transection of the oesophagus is rarely indicated, and has largely been superseded by radiological shunt insertion (e.g. TIPSS).

Answer to Question 22
D

It is likely that this patient is bleeding from oesophageal varices caused by alcohol-induced portal hypertension. Terlipressin reduces the likelihood of continued bleeding by reducing portal pressure and may be helpful prior to endoscopy, or as an adjunct to endoscopic therapy.

Intravenous omeprazole reduces the likelihood of peptic ulcer re-bleeding after endoscopic therapy, but there is no evidence to support its use as an empirical therapy before endoscopy or in the management of variceal haemorrhage. Tranexamic acid is an antifibrinolytic and has been shown to slightly reduce mortality following peptic ulcer haemorrhage in one meta-analysis, while intravenous ranitidine has no impact on outcome of upper GI bleeding from any source. Propranolol is helpful in the primary and secondary prevention of variceal haemorrhage but has no role in the acute setting.

Answer to Question 23
D

Optic atrophy suggests a diagnosis of demyelination. A clear-cut sensory level classically occurs with cord compression, and ankle weakness with saddle area sensory loss would point towards a cauda equina lesion (always examine the saddle area!). In Guillain-Barré syndrome (GBS) there are often cardiovascular abnormalities reflecting autonomic dysfunction. These can be a major problem, manifesting as extreme hypertension or hypotension, tachycardia and bradycardia, and most dramatically as sudden death. In GBS the weakness is greater distally.

Answer to Question 24
E
She has no signs of infection and is not clinically constipated. There is no history of alcohol abuse and there would often be a biochemical or haematological pointer to high alcohol intake such as abnormal liver function tests or raised MCV. Benzodiazepine withdrawal can present with acute confusion and is the most likely explanation in this case.

Answer to Question 25
C
Corticosteroids reduce the duration of a relapse, including optic neuritis, but have no effect on the disease progression or frequency of relapses. Short courses of oral or intravenous methylprednisolone have been shown to be equally effective. Avascular necrosis is a recognised side effect.

Answer to Question 26
D
This presentation is typical of Wernicke–Korsakoff syndrome, caused by thiamine deficiency, most often seen in alcoholics, but to be considered in all patients with malnutrition. The features are confusion, ataxia, ophthalmoplegia and nystagmus. The neurological signs do tend to improve with 3 days of parenteral thiamine, but there are often residual memory problems. CT of the head is likely to be normal. An MRI may show evidence of neuronal loss and demyelination in the midbrain structures.

Answer to Question 27
C
Abnormal blood clotting following paracetamol overdose is a good early marker of synthetic liver function. The INR rises first because Factor VII has the shortest half-life, but it is unusual to see any abnormality in blood clotting less than 18 hours from ingestion, so normal INR at 4 hours is unhelpful. An abnormal INR at the time of admission may indicate chronic liver disease, warfarin ingestion or suggest that ingestion of the drug occurred earlier than the patient reports.

Activated charcoal is only likely to be beneficial if given within 1 hour of ingestion of paracetamol.

If the patient complains of tinnitus, this suggests concurrent salicylate consumption, which requires specific treatment according to the plasma level.

Hepatic encephalopathy rarely occurs less than 48 hours from consumption of paracetamol, and reduction in level of consciousness before this is usually a result of concurrent consumption of alcohol, sedative drugs or hypoglycaemia.

Answer to Question 28
C
Thrombolysis probably improves the outcome of patients with large pulmonary emboli (PE) and signs of right heart failure. Thrombolysis removes the clot obstructing the large pulmonary arteries as well as any clot in the pelvic or deep leg veins. It also reduces the release of serotonin and other neurohumoral factors that tend to exacerbate pulmonary hypertension. Contraindications to thrombolysis include recent surgery, trauma and intracranial pathology.

D-dimer is useful as a negative predictor: patients at low risk of PE and with a normal D-dimer level do not require further investigation and can be reassured, but a high D-dimer level is not helpful as a measure of the size of an embolus.

Answer to Question 29
D
DKA is associated with a high anion gap acidosis.

Answer to Question 30
C
Beta blocker overdose may cause dizziness, hypotension, syncope and heart failure. Bradycardia is a common feature of significant overdose and should be treated by the administration of atropine. Intravenous glucagon may also be given, particularly in patients with haemodynamic compromise. Temporary cardiac pacing may be necessary in patients unresponsive to drug therapy.

Answer to Question 31
E
The working diagnosis must be meningococcal meningitis and the woman must be given an appropriate antibiotic (e.g. cefotaxime 2 g) intravenously without delay. In the very old or immunocompromised it would be appropriate to add ampicillin 2 g six-hourly to cover Listeria, and aciclovir (10 mg/kg eight-hourly, with dose reduction in renal failure) should also be given if herpes simplex encephalitis is a possibility.

Answer to Question 32
D
The history clearly suggests anaphylaxis and treatment with intramuscular epinephrine (0.5 ml of 1/1000) is required. In extremis, epinephrine can be given intravenously, but at reduced dosage: make a 1/10 000 solution

(by diluting 1 ml of 1/1000 to 10 ml with 0.9% saline) and give this at 1 ml/min (0.1 mg/min) until a response has been obtained (or a total of 0.5 mg—5 ml—has been given).

Answer to Question 33

C

The options to be considered, prior to temporary transvenous pacing, in this context are:
• Atropine 0.5–1.0 mg intravenous bolus, repeated as required.
• Isoprenaline, intravenous infusion at 2–10 μg/min.
• External cardiac pacing.

Answer to Question 34

A

The working diagnosis must be opioid overdose, the treatment for which is intravenous naloxone (0.4 mg), repeated up to a total dose of 2 mg depending on clinical response. The half-life of naloxone is shorter than that of opioids, hence if this man wakes up it can be anticipated that he will 're-narcose'. Repeated doses on naloxone may be required; sometime a naloxone infusion is necessary.

Answer to Question 35

E

The base excess is a figure calculated by many blood gas machines to aid interpretation of data. The principles of the calculation are as follows: predict the pH that would arise in normal blood in the presence of the pCO_2 actually measured; then calculate the amount of base that would have to be added to the blood to change the calculated pH into the pH as actually measured. This value is the base deficit or excess, in mmol/l, which quantifies the metabolic component of acid-base disturbance.

Renal failure causes metabolic acidosis with compensatory respiratory alkalosis. In this man the predicted pH (on the basis of measured pCO_2 3.2 kPa) would be alkalotic, and base would have to be removed from the blood to change this to the acidotic value actually measured (pH 7.12). This is expressed as a NEGATIVE base excess.

Answer to Question 36

D

A normal or elevated pCO_2 in an asthmatic indicates failing respiratory effort, and although this woman's oxygen saturation is not severely depressed she is in danger of decompensation and—aside from high flow oxygen, nebulised salbutamol and ipratropium, and steroids—it would be prudent to inform the ICU of her existence. The gases are not bad enough, however, to suggest that cardio-respiratory arrest is imminent.

Pneumothorax must be excluded in any asthmatic, but the presence or absence of pneumothorax can never be inferred from arterial blood gas analysis.

Answer to Question 37

C

Beta2-agonists are pulmonary vasodilators as well as bronchodilators. Their administration can rapidly worsen the V/Q mismatch that is the cause of hypoxia in asthma and they can therefore cause reduction in arterial oxygen tension unless supplemental oxygen is given. This man should be given the highest inspired oxygen concentration that can be obtained. It would also be reasonable to mix ipratropium bromide (500 μg) with the salbutamol given in option C.

Answer to Question 38

A

The European Resuscitation Council guidelines for adult Advanced Life Support suggest that—after Basic Life Support and a precordial thump (if appropriate)—VF/VT should be treated with up to three defibrillation shocks, the first two at 200 J and the third at 360 J.

Answer to Question 39

A

Reactions to N-acetyl cysteine (NAC) are well recognised and are not related to hypersensitivity. NAC can almost always be restarted and total dose safely administered after symptomatic treatment. Oral methionine may be an alternative but is definitely second line. IV chlorpromazine would make hypotension worse and should not be given. Withholding treatment and waiting more than 12 hours would expose patient to risk of liver failure.

Answer to Question 40

E

Activated charcoal provides a large area for adsorption of many drugs ingested as an overdose. Examples of agents not adsorbed by activated charcoal include metals (lithium, iron), hydrocarbons and solvents, alcohols, acids and alkalis.

The Medical Masterclass series

Clinical Skills

General Clinical Issues

Pain Relief and Palliative Care

Medicine for the Elderly

Emergency Medicine

Infectious Diseases and Dermatology

Infectious Diseases

Cardiology and Respiratory Medicine

Cardiology

Neurology, Ophthalmology and Psychiatry

Neurology

Ophthalmology

Psychiatry

Endocrinology

Nephrology

Rheumatology and Clinical Immunology

Index

Note: page numbers in *italics* refer to figures, those in **bold** refer to tables.